TEACHING LIFETIME SPORTS

TEACHING LIFETIME SPORTS

Lawrence F. Butler

BERGIN & GARVEY
Westport, Connecticut • London

Library of Congress Cataloging-in-Publication Data

Butler, Lawrence F.
   Teaching lifetime sports / Lawrence F. Butler.
      p.   cm
   Includes bibliographical references and index.
   ISBN 0–89789–654–8 (alk. paper)—ISBN 0–89789–655–6 (pbk. : aik. paper)
      1. Physical fitness—Study and teaching.   2. Physical education and training—Study and teach-
ing. I. Title.
GV481.B88   2002
796'.07—dc21   2001025180

British Library Cataloguing in Publication Data is available.

Library of Congress Catalog Card Number: 2001025180
ISBN: 0–89789–654–8
     0–89789–655–6 (pbk.)

First published in 2002

Bergin & Garvey, 88 Post Road West, Westport, CT 06881
An imprint of Greenwood Publishing Group, Inc.
www.greenwood.com

Printed in the United States of America

∞™

The paper used in this book complies with the
Permanent Paper Standard issued by the National
Information Standards Organization (Z39.48-1984).

10 9 8 7 6 5 4 3 2 1

Copyright Acknowledgment

Illustrations in Chapter 10 are reproduced with permission from Terry Laughlin, *Total Immersion: The
Revolutionary Way to Swim Better, Faster, and Easier* (Fireside, 1997).

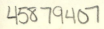

For Audrey, Matthew and Christopher,
and to my parents,
Frank and Helen Butler

Contents

Illustrations

Tables

Preface

Teaching Lifetime Sports was written due to the enormous impact physical activity has on one's health. By focusing on the most popular activities in which a person can participate over the course of his/her lifetime, this book can make a major contribution to the development of the health-related components of physical fitness. As a physical educator, I was driven to create a resource for those teaching lifetime sport activities.

In addition, *Teaching Lifetime Sports* assists teachers in meeting the National Association for Sport and Physical Education's *"Content Standards in Physical Education."* These standards promote the development of a physically educated person. NASPE's definition specifies that a physically educated person:

- Has learned skills necessary to perform a variety of physical activities
- Is physically fit
- Participates regularly in physical activity
- Knows the implications of, and the benefits from, involvement in physical activities
- Values physical activity and its contribution to a healthful lifestyle

This book also serves as a reference for professionals trying to meet the NASPE/NCATE (National Association for Sports and Physical Education/National Association for the Accreditation of Teacher Education) guidelines for physical education teacher preparation. There are nine standards found in the *Guidelines for Teacher Preparation in Physical Education—NASPE/NCATE Guidelines* (4th Edition). This book will cover topics that relate to the following NASPE/NCATE standards:

- Content Knowledge—discipline-specific content and skill knowledge
- Growth and Development—application of growth and development concepts to specific teaching experiences

- Management and Motivation—learning to use a variety of strategies to institute behavior change, manage resources, promote mutual respect and self-responsibility, and motivate students
- Communication—knowledge of effective verbal, nonverbal, and media communication
- Planning and Instruction—pedagogical knowledge and application

Never before have people been more aware of the enormous benefits of physical activity to one's health. These benefits were most recently highlighted in the first "Surgeon General's Report on Physical Activity and Health." This report's most prominent finding was that "people of all ages can improve the quality of their lives through a lifelong practice of moderate physical activity." Although the benefits of lifelong fitness activity are enormous, the United States seems to be experiencing a decline in health-related fitness levels. This downward trend is of particular concern because it is occurring in children as well as adults.

This purpose of this book is to provide practitioners with a single, comprehensive resource that guides them in their efforts to effectively teach the most popular lifetime activities and sports. The information presented will be of particular value to undergraduates in physical education methods classes or those with limited teaching experience for planning, organizing, and sequencing activities. It provides novice teachers with a starting point to effectively teach lifetime sports and fitness activities, and for more experienced teachers, the book will serve as a "one stop shopping" guide for teaching lifetime sports. More importantly, it will assist them in focusing their efforts on sound teaching principles based on current teaching research.

OVERVIEW OF CHAPTERS

Teaching Lifetime Sports is organized into two parts. Part I of the book (Chapters 1–2) provides an introduction to the importance of lifetime fitness activities as well as an overview of the essential skills required to teach them effectively. A review of the declining health- related fitness levels in society today and the inactivity trends in both children and adults sets the stage for the introductory chapter and answers the question "why teach lifetime sports?" Participation in many traditional team sports, often with the primary focus on winning, has often convinced the average student that he/she lacks the skills to participate further. It is here that lifetime sports, both individual and team, can make their greatest contribution to health with a focus on lifetime participation.

Teaching is often described as both an art and a science. Chapter 2 focuses on commonly accepted teaching skills that are applicable to teaching lifetime sports. This review of teaching skills, practices, and strategies is drawn from the most current research pertaining to teaching effectiveness. A basic premise is that student learning is the ultimate goal. This review serves as a foundation which assists both the novice and experienced teacher in focusing on key pedagogical principles prior to planning a particular activity. It proceeds in a logical sequence beginning with considerations in teacher planning through student assessment, and concluding with a review of basic teaching styles and approaches.

Chapter 2 also alerts both novice and experienced teachers to the characteristics of effective teachers noted in recent research. We know that teachers develop their own unique and individual teaching styles and strategies, therefore, this book does not attempt to present a cookbook approach to teaching lifetime sports by listing activities or "tricks of the trade." Rather, it addresses the principles and skills all teachers must develop in order to teach effectively.

Once a foundation for effective teaching has been established, Part II of the book (Chapter 3–10) will focus on specific lifetime activities; allowing the practitioner to become knowledgeable about the particular sports they plan to teach. The key pedagogical principles covered in the first section of the book are integrated, where possible, into each activity. Each chapter concludes with a sample lesson plan, terminology relevant to the activity, and selected readings.

Because rule changes occur frequently, the reader is referred to the national governing bodies of specific sports as well as the National Federation of State High School Associations.

On a more personal note, I hope that this book will not only enhance instruction, but will also have a much broader impact by improving the health and fitness levels of all people.

PART ONE

1

Introduction

IMPORTANCE OF PHYSICAL ACTIVITY IN SOCIETY TODAY

Never before have people been more aware of the enormous benefits of physical activity to one's health. These benefits were most recently highlighted in the first "Surgeon General's Report on Physical Activity and Health" (U.S. Department of Health and Human Services, 1996). This report's most prominent finding was that "people of all ages can improve the quality of their lives through a lifelong practice of moderate physical activity." The benefits of lifelong fitness activities are enormous, yet the United States seems to be experiencing a decline in health-related fitness levels. This downward trend is of particular concern because it is occurring in children as well as adults.

DECLINE IN PHYSICAL FITNESS LEVELS

> The nature of illness that beset our American population has recently undergone a transition of sorts; from a predominance of infectious diseases to the present predominance of degenerative diseases. . . . The increase of such degenerative diseases as cardiovascular accidents (heart attacks and strokes), hypertension, neuroses, and malignancies offers a challenge not only to medicine but to physical education as well. It seems that as improvements in medical science allow us to escape the decimation of such infectious diseases as tuberculosis, diphtheria, poliomyelitis, etc., we live longer, but we fall prey to the degenerative diseases at a slightly later date.
>
> Herbert deVries (1966 p. 244)

This statement by deVries summarizes the challenges we face today to maintain our health through appropriate levels of physical activity. In 1900, infectious diseases such as pneumonia, tuberculosis, and influenza caused one out of every three deaths in the United States. Only 15% of all deaths at the turn of the century were from non-chronic diseases such as heart disease, cancer, and stroke. In the later portion of the twentieth century, however, these statistics drastically changed. By 1994, approximately 60% of all deaths in the United States were attributed to chronic diseases such as cardiovascular disease, cancer, stroke, and bronchitis/emphysema. What has caused this dramatic change? Modern science has clearly been very successful in developing antibiotics and other medical treatments to cure many infectious diseases. Chronic diseases clearly take a long time to develop compared to infectious disease. Infectious diseases killed most people well before the onset of chronic disease. There has been, however, a decrease in the activity levels of many Americans since the 1800s, and this lack of physical activity can contribute to the onset of chronic disease. As technology increased our means of industrial production, more and more people gave up farming and migrated to cities in order to work in factories and offices. Modern day living, with its increased reliance on machines and technology, has significantly increased our sedentary lifestyle and this has contributed to our subsequent health problems.

THE GREAT LEISURE MYTH

The industrial revolution in the nineteenth century, which moved the United States from an agrarian to an industrial society and increased economic prosperity, increased leisure time for some Americans. The growth of cities, a rising standard of living, and the beginning of increased amounts of leisure time were important social forces that combined to promote the growth of sport during this time frame. In addition, working class people won shorter working hours and higher wages, which provided them with greater opportunities to participate in sport (Sage & Eitzen 1993).

During the later half of the twentieth century, however, more and more households had duel breadwinners as women joined the work force in increasing numbers. Leisure time became scarce, and the notion of leisure time became more myth than reality.

TRENDS IN HIGHLY DEVELOPED NATIONS

The following statement on the health benefits of exercise was prepared by a joint Committee of the World Health Organization (WHO) and the International Federation of Sports Medicine (FIMS), and was finalized at a WHO/FIMS meeting on Health Promotion and Physical Activity in Cologne, Germany, on April 7-10, 1994. These organizations encouraged governments around the world to consider the interrelationship of physical activity and health promotion as an important aspect of public health policy.

In the present century mechanization and automation have radically reduced human physical activity. Nowhere has this been more apparent than in highly developed countries, where heavy manual labor has virtually disappeared and labor-saving appliances in homes have drastically reduced physical effort. Increased use of private motor cars and more time spent on sedentary leisure activities, such as television viewing, have to a large extent promoted nonactive lifestyles. Such lifestyles first became prevalent in industrialized countries, but are also increasing in the developing countries. This tendency is not restricted to adults, since there are signs that children and adolescents are also becoming less activity. Lowering of physical activity is thus becoming a world-wide phenomenon.

World Health Organization, 1995

This pattern has become evident in China in recent years. Physical fitness testing has shown that the cardiorespiratory endurance, muscular speed and power, and muscular strength and endurance of urban children in Hong Kong are not as good as their counterparts in Mainland China (Hong, Chan & Li 1998). This information suggests that as countries develop economically, there is a tendency for less physical activity.

PHYSICAL ACTIVITY AND HEALTH—A REPORT OF THE SURGEON GENERAL

This vital report's (U.S. Department of Health and Human Services 1996) findings were numerous but are summarized as follows in its Executive Summary:

Major Conclusions

1. People of all ages, both male and female, benefit from regular physical activity.

2. Significant health benefits can be obtained by including a moderate amount of physical activity (e.g., 30 minutes of brisk walking or raking leaves, 15 minutes of running, or 45 minutes of playing volleyball) on most, if not all, days of the week. Through a modest increase in daily activity, most Americans can improve their health and quality of life.

3. Additional health benefits can be gained through greater amounts of physical activity. People who maintain a regular regimen of activity that is of longer duration or of more vigorous intensity are likely to derive greater benefit.

4. Physical activity reduces the risk of premature mortality in general, and of coronary heart disease, hypertension, colon cancer, and diabetes mellitus in particular. Physical activity also improves mental health and is important for the health of muscles, bones, and joints.

5. More than 60% of American adults are not regularly physically active. In fact, 25% of all adults are not active at all.

6. Nearly half of American youths 12-21 years of age are not vigorously active on a regular basis. Moreover, physical activity declines dramatically during adolescence.

7. Daily enrollment in physical education classes has declined among high school students from 42% in 1991 to 25% in 1995.

8. Research on understanding and promoting physical activity is at an early stage, but some interventions to promote physical activity through schools, worksites, and health care settings have been evaluated and found to be successful.

Physiologic Responses and Long-term Adaptations to Exercise (U.S. Department of Health and Human Services 1996)

1. Physical activity has numerous beneficial physiologic effects. Most widely appreciated are its effects on the cardiovascular and musculoskeletal systems, but benefits on the functioning of metabolic, endocrine, and immune systems are also considerable.

2. Many of the beneficial effects of exercise training from both endurance and resistance activities diminish within 2 weeks if physical activity is substantially reduced, and effects disappear within 2 to 8 months if physical activity is not resumed.

3. People of all ages, both male and female, undergo beneficial physiologic adaptations to physical activity.

Effects of Physical Activity on Health and Disease— Overall Mortality

1. Higher levels of regular physical activity are associated with lower mortality rates for both older and younger adults.

2. Even those who are moderately active on a regular basis have lower mortality rates than those who are least active.

Cardiovascular Disease

1. Regular physical activity or cardiovascular fitness decreases the risk of cardiovascular disease mortality in general, and coronary heart disease mortality in particular. Existing data are not conclusive regarding a relationship between physical activity and stroke.

2. The level of decreased risk of coronary disease attributable to regular physical activity is similar to that of other lifestyle factors, such as not smoking.

3. Regular physical activity prevents or delays the development of high blood pressure, and exercise reduces blood pressure in people with hypertension.

Cancer

1. Regular physical activity is associated with a decreased risk of colon cancer.
2. There is no association between physical activity and rectal cancer. Data are too sparse to draw conclusions regarding a relationship between physical activity and endometrial, ovarian, or testicular cancers.
3. Despite numerous studies on the subject, existing data are inconsistent regarding an association between physical activity and breast or prostate cancers.

Non-Insulin-Dependent Diabetes Mellitus

1. Regular physical activity lowers the risk of developing non-insulin-dependent diabetes mellitus.

Osteoarthritis

1. Regular physical activity is necessary for maintaining normal muscle strength, joint structure, and joint function. In the range recommended for health, physical activity is not associated with joint damage or development of osteoarthritis and may be beneficial for people with arthritis.
2. Competitive athletics may be associated with the development of osteoarthritis later in life, but sports-related injuries are the likely cause.

Osteoporosis

1. Weight-bearing physical activity is essential for normal skeletal development during childhood and adolescence, and maintaining peak bone mass in young adults.
2. It is unclear whether resistance- or endurance-type training can reduce the accelerated rate of bone loss in postmenopausal women in the absence of estrogen replacement therapy.

Falling

1. There is promising evidence that strength training and other forms of exercise in older adults preserve the ability to maintain independent living status and reduce the risk of falling.

Obesity

1. Low levels of activity, resulting in fewer kilocalories used than consumed, contribute to the high prevalence of obesity in the United States.
2. Physical activity may favorably affect body fat distribution.

Mental Health

1. Physical activity appears to relieve symptoms of depression and anxiety, and improves mood.
2. Regular physical activity may reduce the risk of developing depression, although further research is needed on this topic.

Health-Related

1. Physical activity appears to improve health-related quality of life by enhancing psychological well-being, and by improving physical functioning in people compromised by poor health.

Adverse Effects

1. Most musculoskeletal injuries related to physical activity are believed to be preventable by gradually working up to a desired level of activity, and by avoiding excessive amounts of activity.
2. Serious cardiovascular events can occur with physical exertion, but the net effect of regular physical activity is a lower risk of mortality from cardiovascular disease.

Patterns and Trends in the Physical Activity of Adults

1. Approximately 15% of U.S. adults engage regularly (3 times a week for at least 20 minutes) in vigorous physical activity during leisure time.
2. Approximately 22% of adults engage regularly (5 times a week for at least 30 minutes) in sustained physical activity of any intensity during leisure time.
3. About 25% of adults report no physical activity at all in their leisure time.
4. Physical inactivity is more prevalent among women than men, among blacks and Hispanics than whites, among older than younger adults, and among less affluent than more affluent people.
5. The most popular leisure-time physical activities among adults are walking and gardening or yard work.

Adolescents and Young Adults

1. Only about one-half of U.S. young people (ages 12-21 years) regularly participate in vigorous physical activity. One-fourth report no vigorous physical activity.
2. Approximately one-fourth of young people walk or bicycle (i.e., engage in moderate activity) nearly every day.
3. About 14% of young people report no recent vigorous or light-to-moderate physical activity. This indicator of inactivity is higher among females than males and among black females than white females.

4. Males are more likely than females to participate in vigorous physical activity, strengthening activities, and walking or bicycling.

5. Participation in all types of physical activity declines strikingly as age or grade in school increases.

6. Among high school students, enrollment in physical education remained unchanged during the first half of the 1990s, however, daily attendance in physical education declined from approximately 42% to 25%.

7. The percentage of high school students who were enrolled in physical education and who reported being physically active for at least 20 minutes in physical education classes declined from approximately 81% to 70% during the first half of the 1990s.

8. Only 19% of all high school students report being physically active for 20 minutes or more in daily physical education classes.

Understanding and Promoting Physical Activity

1. Consistent influences on physical activity patterns among adults and young people include confidence in one's ability to engage in regular physical activity (e.g., self-efficacy), enjoyment of physical activity, support from others, positive beliefs concerning the benefits of physical activity, and lack of perceived barriers to being physically active.

2. For adults, some interventions have been successful in increasing physical activity in health care settings and at home.

3. Interventions targeting physical education in elementary school can substantially increase the amount of time students spend being physically active in physical education class.

WHAT ARE LIFETIME SPORTS?

There is not any single, commonly accepted definition of lifetime sports. For purposes of this book, and to coincide with the "Surgeon General's report on Physical Activity and Health," lifetime sports are defined as: Those sporting activities that contribute to the health-related components of physical fitness, and that naturally lend themselves to involvement by the average person throughout life.

WHY TEACH LIFETIME SPORTS?

Despite common knowledge that exercise is healthful, more than 60% of American adults are not regularly active, and 25% of the adult population is not active at all. Moreover, although many people have enthusiastically embarked on vigorous exercise programs at one time or another, most do not sustain their participation. Clearly, the processes of developing and maintaining healthier habits are as important to study as the health effects of regular activity on these adults themselves.

In addition to the compelling evidence regarding the enormous benefits of physical activity in the Surgeon General's report, *Healthy People 2000* (1991) is a comprehensive prevention agenda for the nation. The national objectives in *Healthy People 2000* are organized into 22 priority areas, one of which is physical activity and fitness. The natural extension of this program is currently being drafted as *Healthy People 2000: National Health Promotion and Disease Prevention Objectives for the Nation.*

Participating in lifetime sports and activities can contribute significantly to the *Healthy People 2000* objectives for physical activity and fitness which are to:

- "Reduce coronary heart disease deaths
- Reduce overweight prevalence
- Preserve independent functioning in older adults
- Increase moderate physical activity
- Increase vigorous physical activity
- Reduce sedentary lifestyle
- Increase activities that enhance muscular strength, endurance, and flexibility
- Increase sound weight-loss practices
- Increase participation in school physical education
- Increase activity levels in school physical education
- Increase worksite fitness programs
- Increase availability and accessibility of community fitness facilities
- Increase physical activity counseling by primary care providers"

Competitive sporting activities have dominated instruction in physical education and community programs for many years. With all of this instruction occurring, why do so few Americans engage in physical activity? There are a variety of reasons for this trend.

Exercise Versus Physical Activity

Oftentimes, there is an overemphasis on the importance of high-intensity exercise. The National Institute for Health (1995) argues that the "current low rates of regular activity in Americans may be partially due to the misperception of many that vigorous, continuous exercise is necessary to reap health benefits." In addition, the *"no pain—no gain"* mentality has grown in recent years through the media.

Lifetime Sport Philosophy: Overcoming Barriers

Clearly, there is ample evidence to support the need for people of all ages to be physically active. It is essential for people to participate in physical activities that are of interest to them (Slattery 1996). If something is not fun, people will not participate or adhere to a program. For example, it may be difficult to maintain a program of cycling on a stationary bike, however, mountain biking outdoors may significantly increase adherence because it is an adventurous activity.

The appropriate type of activity is best determined by the individual's preferences and what will be sustained (National Institute of Health 1995). The NIH outlines a number of successful approaches for adopting and maintaining a physically active lifestyle. Each person must:

- Perceive a net benefit
- Choose an enjoyable activity
- Feel competent doing an activity
- Feel safe doing an activity
- Be able to easily access the activity on a regular basis
- Be able to fit the activity into the daily schedule
- Feel that the activity does not generate financial or social costs that he or she is unwilling to bear
- Experience a minimum of negative consequences such as injury, loss of time, negative peer pressure, and problems with self-identity
- Be able to successfully address issues of competing time demands
- Recognize the need to balance the use of labor-saving devices (e.g., power lawn mowers, golf carts, automobiles) and sedentary activities (e.g., watching television, use of computers) with activities that involve a higher level of physical exertion

Perceived competence is the best predictor of exercise behavior and adherence in children (Kimiecik, Horn, and Shurin 1996). Children who felt good about their fitness abilities were more likely to participate in the type of moderate-to-vigorous physical activity necessary to improve their health and fitness. The results of this study suggest that children's beliefs were closely related to whether they thought their parents viewed them as competent.

The next chapter will review basic teaching skills and the characteristics of effective teachers. This will provide the novice teacher with a starting point to effectively teach lifetime sports and fitness activities. For more experienced teachers, the upcoming chapter will serve as a "one stop shopping" guide on teaching, and more importantly, will assist them in focusing their efforts on sound teaching principles based on current research.

REFERENCES

Bulletin of the World Health Organization (1995). *73* (2), 135–136.

DeVries, H. (1966). *Physiology of Exercise*. Dubuque, IA: Wm. C. Brown.

Hong, Y., Chan, K.M., & Li, J.X. (1998). Health-related Physical Fitness of School Children in Hong Kong and Mainland China. *Journal of Comparative Physical Education and Sport. 20* (1), 2–10.

Kimiecik, J. C., Horn, T. S., & Shurin, C. S. (1996). Relationships Among Children's Beliefs, Perceptions of their Parents' Beliefs, and their Moderate-to-Vigorous Physical Activity. *Research Quarterly for Exercise and Sport. 67*, 324–336.

National Institute of Health (1995). *NIH Consensus Statement: Physical Activity and Cardiovascular Health. 13* (3).

Public Health Service (1991). *Healthy People 2000: National Health Promotion and Disease Prevention Objectives*. Washington DC: U.S. Government Printing Office. (DHHS Pub. No. PHS 91-50212).

Public Health Service (1996). *Surgeon General's Report on Physical Activity and Health*. Washington, DC: U.S. Government Printing Office.

Sage, G. & Eitzen, D. S. (1993). *Sociology of American Sport*. Dubuque, IA: Brown and Benchmark.

Slattery, M. L. (1996). How Much Physical Activity Do We Need to Maintain Health and Prevent Disease? Different Diseases—Different Mechanisms. *Research Quarterly for Exercise and Sport. 67*, 209–212.

2

Basic Teaching Skills: The Art and Science of Teaching

Teaching has often been described as both an art and a science. Some believe it is an art (Eisner 1983; Highlet 1963) while others have approached it in a more scientific manner (Gage 1963; Siedentop 1983). The artistic-perspective views teaching as dependent on the personal creativity and inspiration of the teacher, including the teacher's artistic approach, inventiveness, intuition, and emotions. The scientific approach can be traced back to John Dewey and his view that learning should be through practice, and trial and error. Siedentop's (1991) text approaches the study of teaching "as if it were a science—that is, amenable to systematic evaluation and capable of being broken down into a series of tasks that can be mastered" (Siedentop 1991, p. 4). However, Siedentop remarks that "it is probably more accurate to define effective teaching as the artistic orchestration of a set of highly developed skills to meet the specific demands of a learning setting" (Ibid.).

What are the specific skills one should develop in order to become a good teacher? A number of physical education textbooks (Graham 1987; Rink 1985; Siedentop 1991) describe a variety of generic teaching skills that a teacher can develop in order to promote student learning. The purpose of this chapter is to alert the reader to the basic teaching skills, competencies, and principles, as described in current physical education literature and research on teaching.

BEFORE WE BEGIN: TEACHER COMMITMENT

Are teachers born or made? This question fuels a debate that is still alive and well today. Although many teachers have an innate aptitude for teaching, everyone can improve upon their teaching skills. Perseverance at being an effective teacher is essential (Siedentop 1995) and this begins with the foundation upon which all other aspects of teaching rest, commitment.

Commitment may be the most important trait that affects teachers' work and, subsequently, their students' achievement (Firestone & Pennell 1993; Reyes 1990). Teacher commitment may be defined as the "psychological identification of the individual teacher with the school and the subject matter or goals, and the intention of that teacher to maintain organizational membership and become involved in the job well beyond personal interest" (Graham 1996, p. 45).

One of the emerging themes in a study on outstanding physical education programs was that the teachers were highly committed (Butler 1993). Teachers in these programs assumed personal responsibility for their professional development, utilized the entire day—including their own personal time—for instruction, continuously thought of ways to add new ideas to their program, and had a great deal of individual interaction with their students. Not only did these teachers tailor their professional development activities to their individual needs, but they initiated their own workshops when none existed. The importance of their "commitment" was evident in these outstanding programs, and the "earned support cycle" in Fig. 2.1 reveals the actual process that occurred.

At least six factors have been identified which influence teacher commitment (Firestone & Pennell 1993; Smylie 1990):

1. Teacher autonomy: the ability of the teacher to determine the procedures to schedule his/her work. The teacher is self-initiating and in control of his/her own actions.
2. Efficacy: the extent to which the teacher believes he/she has the ability to affect student performance.
3. Collaboration: collaborating with another teacher fosters a sense of belonging with the school.
4. Learning opportunities: being involved in professional activities that the teacher perceives as valuable to enhancing his/her effectiveness.
5. Participation in the decision-making process in the school.
6. Feedback about teaching: can enhance a teacher's commitment by confirming the success of some instructional effort.

Graham (1996) has suggested the following strategies to assist teachers in increasing their level of commitment:

1. Be responsive to what your students need from instruction.
2. Become involved with school activities outside the gymnasium. This has the potential to increase your sense of ownership in the organization.
3. Seek out feedback from individuals whose opinions you value.
4. Accept responsibility for your growth as a teacher.

As Graham so aptly reminds us, "developing and maintaining commitment as a teacher is primarily an act of self-empowerment—that is, of accepting responsibility for being the best teacher possible . . . and is the stuff of which real teachers are made" (1996, p. 47).

Figure 2.1   Earned Support Cycle

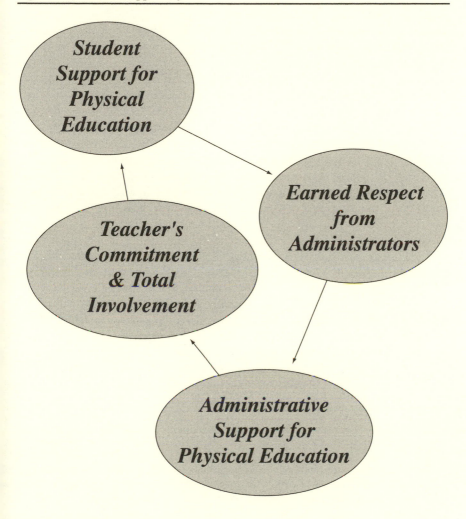

BASIC TEACHING SKILLS

The Importance of Teacher Planning

Proper planning is a vital step in the teaching-learning process. Much of the research on teacher planning has revealed that "teacher planning is an important variable contributing to student achievement" (Stroot & Morton 1989, p. 213) and "good planning is a vital step in the teaching-learning process if we wish to be assured a quality product" (Ibid., p. 222). Studies have revealed that although there are variations in the planning practices of the various teachers in outstanding physical education programs, they all planned extensively and considered it to be essential to the success of their programs (Butler 1993). Teachers in these programs had lessons that were choreographed to the minute, extensive assessment procedures, planned progressions, safety considerations, and cognitive outcomes (Ibid.). From a practical perspective, planning is the "time when teachers sit down with paper and pen in hand, draw upon both past experience and current knowledge in the field, and carefully formulate curriculum, unit, and lesson plans" (Placek 1984, p. 39).

Tyler's (1949) four-step planning model has been taught to pre-service teachers for many years. This model, which has been referred to as an ends-means model, consists of ordering objectives, selecting learning experiences based upon the objectives, organizing the activities to optimize learning, and selecting procedures to evaluate the achievement of the objectives. A number of studies, however, have found that many teachers do not follow Tyler's four step planning model. For example, Zahorik (1975) found that 81% of the teachers simply listed the activities and 70% listed the content (subject matter) as their primary concern when planning. Similarly, Goc-Karp and Zakrajsek (1987) found that teachers focused on the activity or content with little emphasis on skill levels, learning objectives, or evaluation. Other studies (Clark & Yinger 1979; Mann 1975; Merriman 1976; Smith 1977; Taylor 1970; Yinger 1978) have also determined that objectives are not the first item considered by teachers when planning. Placek (1984) found that physical education teachers' lesson plans did not follow the traditional guidelines taught in undergraduate programs, and that student behavior and practical concerns were the primary factors that influenced teacher planning.

Why Plan?

There are five primary reasons why teachers plan (Clark & Yinger 1979; Stroot & Morton 1989):

- To meet personal immediate needs such as anxiety reduction and confidence building
- To learn the material and to collect and organize materials
- To assure that a progression is followed both within and between lessons
- To help him/her stay on-task and to use time as planned
- To fulfill a building or district policy

Types of Planning

There are at least eight different types of planning that teachers may engage in, including weekly, daily, short-range, long-range, yearly, term, unit, and lesson (Yinger 1977; Clark & Yinger 1979). Planning is normally conducted for a school year or semester, for a particular unit or activity, and daily. Physical Education textbooks (Mosston 1986; Graham 1987; Siedentop 1991) offer detailed descriptions of various yearly, unit, and individual lesson planning methods.

Does Teacher Planning Change Over Time?

Teacher planning appears to change dramatically during a teacher's career. Several studies (Stroot & Morton 1989; Cruz 1991; Housner & Griffey 1985) have shown that there are significant differences in the way experienced and beginning teachers plan. Stroot and Morton (1989) found that beginning teachers generally relied on written plans to a greater degree than experienced teachers. As the teachers' experience increased, their plans were used as a review rather than as a rigid script. A study by Cruz (1991) indicated that, when planning, beginning teachers were most concerned with student safety, student enjoyment, the amount of time available, and the availability of equipment. These beginning teachers also changed their planning practices and moved from detailed lesson plans to simply outlining the activities to be covered in class. The reasons given for this change in practice were that planning was not required on the part of the school, planning was time consuming, the use of the facilities was unpredictable, and the beginning teachers did not have a role model to follow who planned. Housner and Griffey (1985) found that experienced teachers were concerned with managing activities during instruction and providing information to facilitate skill acquisition. Inexperienced teachers focused first on student interest, then student involvement, and finally on student performance.

Planning Enhances Student Motivation

The many motivational theories in education can be categorized into two main areas, internal variables and external variables (Placek 1984). Internal variables refer to the students—their perceptions, attitudes, self-concepts, abilities, and values. The external variables refer to the environment of the class itself—such items as teacher behavior, other students, daily class structure, and the program structure (Ibid., p. 27).

Physical Education classes are often plagued by a lack of interest on the part of students, and teachers have their share of students who do not dress out for class or who utilize medical excuses to avoid class (Placek 1984). There are many possible reasons for this lack of interest, and physical education teachers do have strategies to motivate the students in their classes. Placek suggests that teachers examine the perceptions of individual students. From these examinations, the teacher may learn that a student was injured in a previous activity and therefore avoids class, the student's parents may not value physical activity, or the student may be embarrassed due to a lack of skill or fitness. By demonstrating interest and compassion for students, the teacher may be able to improve participation levels.

The interactions that teachers have with their students are very important. Quarterman (1977) described the teaching behavior of 24 K-8 physical education teachers and found that 85% of all their feedback interactions with students were negative or corrective in nature. Teachers need to be aware of this syndrome and insure that their comments are positive in nature. In fact, Siedentop (1976) recommends maintaining a ratio of four to one positive to negative comments.

Teachers need to examine not only their own interactions with students, but also their daily class structure, overall program structure, and the activity choices students have in order to maximize student interest (Placek 1984).

Goal setting is another technique that teachers can use to enhance student motivation (Boyce 1989; Pemberton & McSweigin 1989). Boyce found that students with established performance goals tend to perform better on tasks and skills than those who were told to "do their best" (1989, p. 22). Performance goals are most effective when they are objective, measurable, specific, short in duration, meaningful to the student, individualized, and set at an appropriate level of difficulty (Ibid.).

Harter's (1978; 1981) competence motivation theory suggests that there are four indirect methods for increasing student motivation: (1) the degree of success experienced by the students; (2) the level of task difficulty; (3) the feedback received; (4) student perceptions of control in a situation. In general, the more successful students are in performing a task, the greater their motivation. Skills that match students' ability levels, yet challenge them, maintain their motivational level. Providing students with a perception that they have control is also an essential component. Tjeerdsma (1995, p. 38) has summarized some of the key aspects of developing the students' perception of control:

- Let students choose the type of equipment they use (junior size basketball or regulation size; volleyball trainer or regulation volleyball)
- Let students choose their own partners/groups (the need to choose someone with whom they can work productively should be emphasized)
- Let students decide whether to keep score during games
- Give students a choice of participating in either competitive or cooperative games
- Allow students to choose whether they will participate in a tournament
- Use teaching by invitation (Graham, et al. 1993) in which alternative tasks are presented to the entire class and then students choose a task they will perform. ("You may start your game with a serve or a toss over the net"; "You may want to continue passing and catching as we have just done, or you may want to add a defender")

The importance of student choice as an important consideration to promote student motivation has been confirmed by Mancini, Cheffers, and Rich (1983) who cited a group of studies which found that students had a more favorable attitude toward an activity when they were offered a choice.

Lesson Plans

As a general guide, when formulating lesson plans, it is recommended that a teacher take into account:

- learning objectives
- class size
- frequency of class meetings
- equipment and facilities
- personal characteristics of the students

- students' skill level and interests
- organization of students and the environment
- activities or lesson focus
- student evaluation, and evaluation/critique of the lesson

Summary: Key Points on Teacher Planning for Lifetime Sports

- Proper planning, at the yearly, unit, and daily level is a vital and necessary step for effective teaching
- When planning, take into account:
  - learning objectives
  - equipment and facilities
  - organization of the students and the teaching environment
  - specific activities, progressions, or lesson focus
  - student assessment
  - assessment/critique of the lesson
- Beginning teachers or teachers involved in a new activity for the first time need to plan more extensively
- Demonstrating interest and compassion for students can enhance their interest
- Focus on providing "positive" feedback to enhance student motivation. Provide at least a ratio of four to one positive to negative/corrective comments
- Provide students with as many choices as possible to enhance motivation
- Establish performance goals to enhance student motivation which are:
  - Objective
  - Measurable
  - Specific
  - Short in duration
  - Meaningful to the student
  - Individualized
  - Set at an appropriate level of difficulty in order to achieve an 80% success rate

Developing Course Content

Rink defined content development as "teaching stripped of its managerial concerns" and the "manner in which the teacher manipulates the content so that learning can occur" (1995, p. 98). Effective teachers go through a process in developing content. The process components of content development in physical education are called extension, refinement, and application (Ibid.).

- *Extension* communicates a concern for changing the complexity or difficulty of student performance.
- *Refinement* communicates a concern for the quality of student performance.
- *Application* communicates a concern for moving the student focus from how to do the movement to how to use the movement. The purpose of this process is to have the student move from one level of performance to another.

Teachers often make many sequencing decisions based on information such as student interest, motivation, success, and enjoyment (Petersen 1991). Other

Figure 2.2   Optimal Planning Cycle

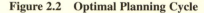

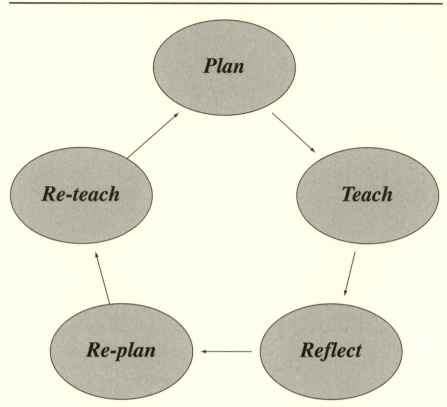

factors, such as the practical aspects of the schedule, the weather, and the facility, also affect sequencing decisions. Cruz (1991) found that for beginning teachers the most important considerations in developing content were that the activities had to be adequate for the amount of time they had with their classes, that the equipment required was available to them, and that the students were safe and had fun.

In addition, linking is an important concept in developing the course content and lesson content. If it doesn't make sense, the behavior problems will increase.

Effectively Presenting Material

Rosenshine and Stevens (1986) have summarized the work of researchers on the characteristics of effectively presenting new material in general education. This summary serves as a good guideline for teaching new psychomotor skills as well.

Aspects of Clear Presentations

1. Clarity of Goals and Main Points
   a. State the goals or objectives of the presentation
   b. Focus on one point at a time
   c. Avoid digressions
   d. Avoid ambiguous phrases

2. Step-by-step presentations
   a. Present the material in small steps
   b. Organize the material so that one point is mastered before the next point is given
   c. Give explicit, step-by-step directions
   d. Present an outline when the material is complex

3. Specific and concrete procedures
   a. Model the skill
   b. Give detailed and redundant explanations for difficult points

4. Check for students' understanding
   a. Be sure that students understand one point before moving on to the next point
   b. Ask the students questions to monitor their comprehension of what has been presented
   c. Have students summarize main points in their own words
   d. Review the parts that students are having difficulty with, either by further teacher explanation or by students tutoring other students.

Presenting new material may be subdivided into two categories; modeling (demonstrating) and providing instructional cues (key teaching phrases).

Modeling: A Picture's Worth a Thousand Words

One of the most effective methods in teaching is modeling, better known as demonstrating. It can be a powerful tool for teaching and learning because complex skills can be better understood by students through seeing the performance. "Modeling is a process of teaching through example that produces learning through imitation" (Charles 1985, p. 142). Dauer and Pangrazi remind us that "demonstrations can illustrate variety or depth of movement, show something unique or different, point out items of technique or approach, illustrate different acceptable styles, and show progress" (1989, p. 88). Modeling may be performed by either the teacher or a skilled student in the class. It is often done at the beginning of the class period to give students an overview of the skill and then used several times throughout the lesson to re-emphasize the key teaching points. "Modeling is successful only if it sustains the children's attention" (Sander 1989, p. 14).

Modeling may be even more effective if we use the behavior of one student as an example for others to imitate (Siedentop 1983). Students can learn through imitation and often emulate the desired behavior. Whenever possible, students who can demonstrate newly learned skills should be utilized. This can serve to enhance student motivation in general as well as serve as a sign of achievement for the particular student who performed the demonstration.

Summary on Modeling

- Despite its value, teachers often do not take full advantage of modeling
- The demonstration of the skill should be accurate and in the proper sequence
- Demonstrate each component of a skill, or progression, as well as the entire skill several times—a picture is worth a thousand words
- Use a student to demonstrate whenever possible

Providing Instructional Cues

Teachers have a finite amount of time in which to conduct their class, and instructional time is therefore precious. In order to maximize student practice time, teachers must avoid the common error of talking too much during the instructional phase. Effective teachers choose their words carefully in order to communicate their essential teaching points. Instructional cues may be thought of as the "key phrases" teachers use to communicate the critical aspects of a movement skill or task to the performer (Rink 1985). They may also be thought of as the "words that quickly and efficiently communicate to the learner the proper technique and performance of skills or movement tasks" (Dauer and Pangrazi 1989, p. 86). Teachers should be cautious of providing too many ideas and concepts that can lead to "information overload" and overwhelm a student when they are attempting a new skill. When used properly, instructional cues can greatly assist the student in focusing on the most important aspects involved in learning a new skill.

When developing instructional cues, Dauer and Pangrazi (1989) suggest that they be precise, short, integrated, and action-oriented. In order to save time, Siedentop (1991) recommends that instructional cues be embedded in the environment via posters, pictures, and diagrams so they are there for students when they need them. Posters using cue words can be placed throughout the learning area describing the key elements of the skill being taught.

Use of Metaphors

Teachers can use "metaphors" as instructional cues to enhance student enthusiasm, performance, and ultimately student learning. Metaphors may be defined as "a way of speaking in which one thing is expressed in terms of another, whereby this bringing together throws new light on the character of what is being described" (Gorden 1978). For example, an effective metaphor in teaching racquetball might be, "when playing racquetball, the center court position should be like a magnet" thus conveying to the student that they should always be drawn back to center court after hitting the ball. Metaphors may also increase arousal level, which is advantageous when performing gross motor skills (Oxendine 1970). Gassner (1997) pointed out that metaphors have the advantage of being non-threatening and can bypass the natural resistance to change. Instead of using criticism to teach, meaningful and well-timed metaphors can positively influence a student's efficiency of learning.

Summary: Instructional Cues

- Concise and precise
- Action-oriented
- Thought-out well in advance in order to convey key teaching points
- Where possible, embed in the environment via posters, pictures, and diagrams
- Consider using metaphors as part of your repertoire of instructional cues

Providing Effective Feedback

Teacher feedback has been consistently identified as an essential component of teaching that enhances student learning. Dauer and Pangrazi (1989) contend that "if used properly, it can enhance a student's self-concept, improve the focus of performance, increase the rate of on-task behavior and improve student understanding." Therefore, providing meaningful feedback is an important skill for teachers to develop if student learning is to take place. Feedback may be defined as "information about a response that is used to modify the next response" and "teacher behavior that is in response to student actions" (Siedentop 1991). Others have defined teacher feedback as a "variety of teacher reactions to student behavior, such as teacher praise, correction, and affirmation of a correct response" (Rink 1985).

Feedback interactions can be categorized as either general or specific, and further subdivided as positive, corrective, or negative in nature (Siedentop 1991). Much of the beginning work in describing feedback patterns in physical education found that most teachers gave general praise and specific criticisms (Tobey 1974). Further studies have shown that physical education teachers spend very little time giving feedback to students. Feedback tends to occur at the rate of thirty to sixty events per thirty minutes (Quarterman 1977). General feedback is used more frequently than specific feedback; feedback tends to be more corrective in nature as opposed to positive or negative, and feedback is typically directed toward an individual rather than a group or the class as a whole (Fishman & Tobey 1978).

How to Provide Students with Effective Feedback

Rink (1985) contended that physical education teachers should consider the following factors in giving feedback: to whom is the feedback directed, the specificity of the feedback, the positive or negative aspects of the feedback, the evaluative or corrective aspects of the feedback, the congruency (agreement) of the feedback with the task, and the timing of the feedback. While a teacher can be very positive in providing "corrective" feedback, an overuse of this type can have a chilling effect on the teacher-student relationship.

In order to provide feedback to students, Docheff (1990) has developed a simple, yet effective method for providing meaningful feedback through his "feedback sandwich." The feedback sandwich is comprised of reinforcing, informational, and motivational phrases.

- A *reinforcement* phrase provides the student with a sense that they are heading in the right direction in performing the skill.
- An *information* phrase is the "meat" of the sandwich and provides the critical technical information to improve skill performance.
- A final *motivational* phrase is provided to encourage the student further.

Here is an example of a feedback sandwich statement that a teacher might develop for teaching a ceiling shot in racquetball. Note that all phrases are concise and precise in nature.

1. "You're keeping your eye on the ball well, John!" (reinforcement of an instructional cue).
2. "Now step into the ball a little more as you strike it." (key technical information).
3. "You're on you way to a great ceiling shot!" (encouraging motivational phrase).

The advantage of this method is that it enables the teacher to effectively, yet efficiently, provide feedback to an individual student and move on to another.

Group-directed Feedback

Teachers are often faced with thirty or more students in a class and providing effective, individualized feedback can be a challenge. Teachers may not have sufficient time to observe a single student for several practice attempts, provide them with effective feedback, and then observe them to insure they are now performing the skill correctly. "Group-directed feedback" is a realistic, supplemental method for providing students with effective feedback. To use this approach, the teacher stops student practice momentarily to provide specific feedback that is useful to the entire group. This "group-directed" technique can be particularly effective if combined with a brief teacher or, better yet, student demonstration of the desired movement pattern or skill. The key is to provide the feedback quickly, reinforcing the key cues, in order to allow the students to return to practice. The teacher can repeat this, as necessary, in order to continually provide feedback that enhances learning.

Use of Praise

Students often seek teacher attention, and receiving feedback from a teacher is a source of that attention. Teachers should be aware of how to effectively provide praise. The "quality" of teacher praise is more important than the "frequency," and the following guidelines (Brophy 1981) provide advice on how teachers can use praise effectively. Effective praise:

- Is delivered contingent upon performance
- Specifies the particulars of the accomplishment
- Shows spontaneity, variety, and other signs of credibility
- Should praise genuine progress or accomplishment (quality, credibility, and the individualized nature of the accomplishments are more important than quantity)
- Should be given when students may not realize their accomplishment
- Should be informative or appreciative but not controlling (the task should be on task-relevant aspects, not on pleasing the teacher)
- Should be natural rather than theatrical or intrusive
- Should be private
- Should be individualized
- Should attribute success to effort and ability implying that similar successes can be expected in the future

Teach Students How to Give Feedback

Peer-feedback can be an effective supplement to teacher feedback and promotes "active learning" in the class. It is important to note that placing greater responsibility for learning on the student does not imply a lessened responsibility on the teacher. Rather than passively waiting their turn, students can be encouraged to "coach" one another by reinforcing the "instructional cues" that the teacher has provided. In a golf lesson, for example, the teacher may use the instructional cue "head down" while teaching the basic golf swing. Students can then pair up and focus on this key point when observing one another practice.

Summary: Key Points on Providing Effective Feedback

- Provide students with specific, corrective, and congruent feedback in a positive manner
- Plan and link your feedback statements based on your instructional cues
- Feedback should be immediate
- Keep feedback statements simple. Avoid overloading the student with too much information at once
- Incorporate the "feedback sandwich" for your individualized feedback
- Utilize "group-directed feedback" to provide meaningful feedback to larger classes
- Promote "active learning" by teaching students how to provide feedback to one another (have them reinforce your instructional cues)

Regulating Student Practice

"Mere activity is not enough to assure quality. The activity must be focused, with students engaged in relevant tasks" (Beauchamp, Darst, & Thompson 1990, p. 92). One of the characteristics of effective teachers is that they find ways to keep their students appropriately engaged in the subject matter a high percentage of the available time (Siedentop 1983). In addition to having students on-task a high percentage of the time, there must be an appropriate matching of content to student abilities. High-quality practice time has been associated with greater student achievement in physical education. For example, one study found that the most effective classes spent 22% of their time practicing a skill, while the less effective classes spent only 7.7% of their time practicing the same skill (Pieron 1981). The concept of Academic Learning Time-Physical Education (ALT-PE) maintains that students should not only be engaged in relevant physical education content for a unit of time, but should also be engaged in a way that they are successful at least 80% of the time (Siedentop 1991). McLeish (1985) reached several conclusions concerning the ALT-PE learning model:

- Learning is maximized in direct proportion to the number and type of opportunities to practice
- We learn best by concentrating on practicing the motor, cognitive, or psychomotor skill, by actual doing, or by observing others performing the skill
- There is little advantage to be gained in practicing the skill at a difficulty level which results in a failure rate greater than 10%

Teachers involved in teaching physical activities often spend a great deal of their time imparting instruction, often at the expense of practice. An effective teacher is "one who provides practice that is pertinent, purposeful, progressive, paced, and participatory" (Siedentop 1983, p. 45).

Pacing a Lesson

A strong, smooth pace is very important for effective teaching (Kounin 1970). In general, successful teachers move students briskly step by step, but the steps themselves are small and within the grasp of the students. "Effective lessons have a brisk pace that is not slowed down but maintains its forward momentum, especially during transition and management tasks" (Siedentop 1991, p. 224). Maintaining a brisk pace is also an important factor in preventing behavior problems.

In order to ensure a smooth pace, the teacher must use effective planning and class management techniques. Typically, students spend over 35% of their time in physical education classes waiting (Costello 1977). A brisk pace will help to reduce this waiting time. It is suggested that student-waiting time can be reduced by using equipment efficiently, making rapid transitions between class segments, and structuring lessons to keep students moving (Costello & Laubach 1978).

Providing for Student Safety

Teachers are responsible for providing a safe learning environment for their students. Providing for student safety is defined as the process of structuring the learning environment in such a way as to limit the possibility for physical and emotional harm and providing safety instruction (Doolittle & Girard 1991). Also, teachers must be aware of psychological safety as well as physical safety in their classes (Siedentop 1991). Psychological safety refers to students feeling safe about the activities they are participating in and being free from ridicule and embarrassment. There are some inherent risks associated with physical activities and it is often the goal of a unit or program to teach students how to take appropriate risks. "One of the most important outcomes of a physical education program is its ability to offer students an opportunity to take a risk and overcome fear" (Dauer and Pangrazi 1989, p. 89).

Teachers have a number of strategies they can employ to ensure a safe learning environment for their students. "Whenever a potentially hazardous activity is being undertaken, the teacher should emphasize clearly the rules that have been established with regards to the hazard and that these rules should be described, prompted often, and students should be held accountable for obeying them" (Siedentop 1991, p. 209). Safety procedures should also be taught at the beginning of the school year by introducing them with other general rules and procedures (Graham et al. 1987).

The use of proper lead-up activities and progressions in teaching various skills can improve the level of safety. Students who are taught skills through a series of appropriate progressions will not only develop confidence in their abilities, but will also tend to behave in a safe manner (Siedentop 1991). In addition, it is critical that safety inspections be conducted by the teacher at regular intervals in order to maximize safety (Dauer & Pangrazi 1989).

Monitoring/Active Supervision

Monitoring can be defined in several ways. Siedentop defined monitoring as "the informal and formal ways of observing and assessing the degree to which student performance meets specifications" (1991, p. 218). Anderson defined it as "silently attending to students who are performing motor activities" (1980, p. 40). Informal monitoring refers to the active supervision by the teacher in which the teacher responds to task accomplishments and corrects task errors (Siedentop 1991). Formal monitoring usually involves a task check list which produces a record of a student's performance relative to the instructional task. Physical education teachers also use monitoring for student rewards and incentives.

Another important safety concept is that of "active supervision," in which the teacher responds positively to task accomplishments and corrects task errors (Siedentop 1991). Active supervision helps to prevent students from straying off-task to activities in which they may be injured. Barrette (1977) found that physical education teachers spent 21.1% of their class time silently monitoring student performance of motor activity.

Monitoring is undertaken in physical education in order to determine if learning objectives are being met. Without a monitoring system in place, teachers would not have a way of knowing if they were teaching effectively. Monitoring is also the mechanism for gathering information in preparation for giving feedback.

Providing Effective Closure to a Lesson

Siedentop defined closure as "the end-of-class time when teachers bring together the parts of a lesson to make it whole for students, to make sure students understood the important elements learned in the lesson, to reestablish the importance of the elements, and to assess and validate students' feelings relative to the lesson" (1991, p. 222).

Several authors (Jensen 1988; Marks 1988) have offered teachers guidelines to follow in order to have an effective closure to their classes. They include: (1) students should be made aware of what was accomplished in the lesson; (2) closure is an opportunity for student recognition; (3) it is an opportunity to check students feelings; (4) it can be a review; and (5) it serves as a transition from intense activity to classroom behavior. Typically this time period takes only two to three minutes in physical education (Graham 1987).

Class Management

The studies of Academic Learning Time in Physical Education (ALT-PE) indicated that students spent 15-22% of their time in management activities, and that managerial and organizational skills are the largest part of the explanation for the small amounts of learning time (McLeish 1985, Siedentop 1983). Class management time will also vary depending on the activity. McLeish (1985) found that management time in swimming was 14% and 32% in gymnastics, while Chung (1985) found that fitness classes spent 7% of their time in management tasks.

Instructional and student practice times are a teacher's precious commodities. "Class management is considered central to the task of teaching" (Doyle 1986, p. 394). Its purpose is to make instructional time more efficient (Sander 1989). Class management may be defined as "the ability of the teacher to organize the learning environment and maintain appropriate behavior" (Rink 1985, p. 270). Nichols (1990) describes effective class management as the procedures for getting the class started, giving meaningful instructions, securing and putting away equipment, organizing and moving the class throughout the lesson, and planning closure for the lesson. Nichols contends that effective management is essential if learning is to be maximized.

Kounin (1977) described three characteristics of effective class managers. They are withitness, desist clarity, and overlappingness. These characteristics focus on using preventative techniques, as opposed to dealing with misconduct after it occurs. "Withitness" refers to the teacher's ability to know what is going on and to target misbehavior accurately and with good timing. "Withit" teachers notice misbehavior early before it spreads and are accurate in reprimanding the originator rather than an innocent bystander. "Desist clarity" refers to the teacher's ability to give specific feedback on behavior. "Overlappingness" is the teacher's ability to handle several things simultaneously with a smooth, uninterrupted flow of events. Clearly the image projected here is that of the "teacher as ringmaster."

There are a number of effective strategies to improve class management techniques. By learning to obtain and hold children's attention, by managing behavior, and by using effective organizational techniques, time for instruction, activity, and feedback can be maximized (Sander 1989). In order to promote effective class management, the followings strategies are suggested (Nichols 1990):

- Establish a class routine
- Establish a signal for students to listen
- Get off to a good start by beginning class promptly
- Get the class involved in an activity quickly
- Give instructions which are short and to the point
- Keep the lesson pace moving
- Maximize student participation
- Plan student groupings in advance
- Plan for the transitions from activity to activity

Effective teachers spend less time organizing their students during class, provide more practice time, maximize the use of equipment, and transition students from one activity to another efficiently (Phillips & Carlisle 1983). From a practical perspective, "successful managers 'hover' over activities at the beginning of the year and usher them along until students have learned the system" (Doyle 1986, p. 412).

Behavior Management

Behavior management is a subcategory of class management (Sander 1989) and studies of this type comprise the largest body of class management literature in physical education (Luke 1989). Effective behavior management techniques are essential in order to develop and maintain an environment conducive to learning. Jansma, French, and Horvak stated that the "best physical educators are the best behavioral engineers" and that "behavioral engineering is an essential skill for physical educators" (1984, p. 80). Earls found that "the absence of discipline and motivation problems is conspicuous in classes of distinctive teachers" (1981, p. 64). The lack of discipline in some schools has been identified as an important concern of parents, teachers, and administrators (Gallup 1984; 1986).

There are several preventative strategies offered to assist teachers in managing student behavior. Graham et al. (1987) recommends five techniques to enhance appropriate student behavior:

- Positive student-teacher interactions
- Ignoring inappropriate student behavior

- Nonverbal interactions such as physical proximity to the student in question
- Eliminating differential treatment of students
- Person to person dialogue away from the class setting

Student Assessment

Safrit (1986) defined assessment as the use of measurement data to make both a diagnosis and prescription for student learning, as well as to evaluate how much is learned. Veal (1988) identified three phases of assessment in physical education; preassessment, which should be used in planning; formative assessment, which should be used in teaching and learning; and summative assessment, which should be used for evaluation.

There is a wide gap between pupil assessment theory and practice. Inservice teachers do not use the assessment practices that they were taught in professional preparation courses. Kneer's (1986) study regarding the use of evaluation procedures in secondary physical education yielded some interesting results. Twenty-four % of the teachers said they did not believe in using evaluation theory, 16% said it takes too much time, and 40% said it was not necessary. Veal (1988) found that many teachers felt that the techniques they learned in their teacher-education courses were not practical in their teaching situations. Other pupil assessment studies have shown that teachers primarily appraise student participation, effort, and attitude rather than achievement of skills (Austin & Wilhelm 1986; Carre et al. 1983; Imwold et al. 1982; Kneer 1986; Loughrey 1975). Some authors (Imwold et al. 1982; Locke & Dodds 1981) contend that part of the problem is inadequate preparation in the professional preparation programs.

In an age where accountability is becoming ever more important, physical education teachers must utilize effective assessment techniques. The challenge is to devise efficient, simple, and reliable ways to measure and record improvement, and then to teach those techniques to teachers (Veal 1988).

TEACHING STYLES AND APPROACHES

Direct Instruction

Often referred to as "active teaching" (Rosenshine 1979), direct instruction is the most predominant style of teaching in physical education today (Siedentop 1991). Direct instruction is a "holistic term that implies a teaching-learning environment with the following characteristics; it is a task orientated but relaxed environment with a focus on goals, there is a high degree of monitoring of student progress toward these goals, the activities are structured, and there is immediate feedback" (Rink 1985, p. 269). This style places a great deal of emphasis on student accountability, focused learning, and active teaching (Rink 1985). In this style, the students are searching for the right answer that the teacher is looking for (Mosston 1981).

When the achievement of basic skills is the goal, direct instruction does have an advantage over more learner-centered styles in terms of student learning (Peterson 1979). "Part of the success of active teaching can be attributed to the organizational and supervisory aspects of the format that allow teachers to manage student engagement" (Siedentop 1991, p. 229).

Cohort Instruction

Cohort instruction is one of the most common teaching styles in physical education today and may be defined as a completely teacher-directed style with all students working on the same skill at the same time and progressing at the same rate. Advocates of this style of instruction believe that the class is unduly disrupted if the teacher attempts to meet the individual needs of the students. This style will tend to work best when teaching students of the same ability level. The disadvantage of this style is that the individual needs of the students are not met.

Individualized Instruction

The individualized style is based on the concept of student-centered learning through an individualized curriculum (Dauer & Pangrazi 1989, p. 94). In this style, each student's needs are assessed and an individual plan is established with specific behavioral objectives. A wide array of teaching strategies are utilized so that the students may progress at their own rate (Dauer & Pangrazi 1989). The teacher sets up the learning environment which allows the student to control the rate of learning and to receive individual feedback about progress.

Contracting

Contracting is "a form of individualized instruction in which students sign a learning contract to complete a sequence of learning tasks according to a predetermined set of criteria" (Siedentop 1991, p. 240). This self-instructional format may take place within the school setting or at a local site without the teacher's presence. Contract teaching requires more effort on the part of the teacher (Morton 1989) for planning, organizing, and tracking of student progress than the more traditional teaching styles do. The actual written contract is very specific in nature and covers such topics as: the learning tasks to be completed, the amount of practice time required, and the performance criteria required for various grades (Siedentop 1991). Although it may require more effort, contract teaching can be "an effective instructional style that can motivate and renew excitement in physical education for students and teachers alike" (Morton 1989, p. 13).

Learning Center Format

Learning center format, also referred to as "station teaching," is an alternative to teaching a class as a whole (Graham et al. 1987). In this format, the teacher divides the students into small groups utilizing several different areas of the teaching space. This allows two or more tasks to go on simultaneously. The students work on different activities at each learning center and rotate from station to station either systematically or at their own discretion. The teacher monitors the stations offering encouragement, feedback, and insuring that the pace of the lesson is maintained (Rink 1985). The teacher can individualize instruction using this format because the learning centers can be set up so students of varying ability levels can work on related skills. The teacher can write task descriptions at each learning center to further reduce the time spent instructing (Graham et al. 1987). This is important because it has been found that students often spend as much as 35% of their time in physical education classes waiting (Costello 1977). The advantage of this style is that student-waiting time is reduced due to the number of stations. "Many teachers choose station teaching as a teaching strategy because if offers flexibility in content selection and all students can be active doing different things" (Rink 1985, p. 199).

Peer/Reciprocal Teaching

Peer teaching, also known as reciprocal teaching (Mosston 1966), is an instructional format in which peers play an active role in the learning process (Siedentop 1991). It is an instructional strategy that transfers the teacher's responsibility for instructional components to the student (Rink 1985). The teacher's primary role is to plan, and then monitor, the tutoring process. As the size of a learning group gets smaller, achievement increases with one-on-one tutoring having the greatest effect (Cooke, Heron, & Heward 1983; Bloom 1983). In the peer/reciprocal teaching style, the students typically work in small groups of two to three and assume the instructional role. The advantages of this format are that: the tutors benefit from having to teach to their peers; instruction is more individualized; groups can progress at their own pace; greater feedback produces a higher number of correct responses; and students learn more responsibility by acting as tutors. This format requires more time and energy in the planning process with the key to success being the working relationships between the students (Siedentop 1991).

Problem Solving

Problem solving involves the presentation of a task requiring a verbal or movement solution determined through movement responses (Rink 1985). The problem solving style involves input, reflection, choice, and response (Dauer and Pangrazi 1989). In this approach, cognitive goals are often more important than motor-skill and strategy goals (Siedentop 1991, p. 232), and the teacher structures the problem so that there is more than one possible answer. Problems can be designed to be simple for young children and more complex for older children, while solutions can involve an individual or partner approach. Dauer and Pangrazi (1989) identify the five-step process for implementing this style. The problem is (1) presented to the students, (2) procedures are determined, (3) students experiment and explore possible solutions, (4) students observe, evaluate, and discuss the solutions, and (5) the students refine and expand their solutions. The problem solving style can be used to teach physical education concepts, relationships, strategies, and the proper use of skills for specific solutions (ibid.).

Guided Discovery

Guided discovery is a "teacher-controlled style in which a carefully arranged series of instructions gradually leads the student through a series of experiences in which a goal is finally reached" (Siedentop 1983, p. 169). "The cumulative effect of this sequence, a convergent process, leads the learner to discover the sought concept, principle, or idea" (Mosston 1986, p. 170). This style of teaching is therefore used most often with young students (grades K-3) in movement-oriented lessons that focus on space, time, and force.

Reflective Teaching

Reflective teaching is not a specific style of teaching but rather a process by which teachers assess their own teaching. Graham et al. defined reflective teaching as "employing a variety of teaching skills that interact effectively with the particular teaching environment" (1987, p. 6). Effective teaching, according to Graham et al., is situational rather than generic. A packaged teaching method that works in one school setting may not work well when transplanted to another. A reflective teacher is "one who can design and implement an educational program that is congruent with the idiosyncrasies of a particular school situation" (ibid.). The following variables are most often mentioned to illustrate the need for reflective teaching (ibid.):

- Socioeconomic status of the children
- Size of the classes
- Teacher's education and experience
- Equipment and facilities
- Subject matter
- Discipline

Anderson reminds us of the importance of analyzing and reflecting on one's teaching and that "the analysis of teaching is not a convenient adjunct to teaching; it is teaching" (1980, p. 2). Stagnation may be the result if teachers do not reflect and analyze their own teaching.

An Eclectic Approach

Teachers may choose one particular style or they may elect to use a combination of several styles. This can be a very effective approach. For example, in teaching racquetball, the teacher may utilize direct instruction at the beginning of class to present new material and then switch to a peer-reciprocal style when the students begin practicing the skills.

CHARACTERISTICS OF EFFECTIVE TEACHERS

What makes a good teacher? This appears to be such a simple question. We know when we have had a good teacher yet it is often difficult to describe them. We have all had teachers who seem to have something special that sets them apart from all the rest. For purposes of this chapter, "effective teachers" are those who demonstrate the teaching skills that promote "student learning." Teaching is a complex activity. It has many components and cannot be reduced to a single element or even a small group of elements. "Successful teaching involves the orchestration of a complex set of variables and only a few of these variables have been identified consistently through teaching research" (Pieron & Graham 1984). Effective instruction involves selecting from a large repertoire and orchestrating those teaching behaviors that are appropriate to a specific situation and group of students (Brophy & Good 1986).

As a starting point, one professor of the year suggests that "good teachers really want to be good teachers" (Beidler 1997) and Siedentop (1995) reminds us that "teachers who are effective, persevere at being effective."

The material presented in this section is not meant to be prescriptive. It is not intended to simply provide a cookbook approach to teaching with proven "recipes for success." Rather, its intent is to alert those who wish to improve their teaching to some of the findings on teacher effectiveness. It is only through effective teaching that we can impart the full benefits of lifetime sports for our students.

Brophy & Good (1986) have identified a number of key areas that good teachers focus on such as role definition, expectations, and time allocation. These teachers:

- Emphasize instruction
- Communicate high expectations; expect students to master the curriculum; have a "can do" attitude, perceiving their students as capable of learning the material and themselves as capable of teaching it to them effectively. These teachers set higher goals than other teachers, and they are more persistent in laboring to meet those goals and overcoming obstacles if necessary (Brophy & Evertson 1976)
- Allocate sufficient time to curricular activities
- Focus on class management
- Have high student-engaged time
- Consistent success/academic learn time
- Engage students in activities that are appropriate in difficulty level

The Art of Teaching

A distinctive teacher is one who stands out from the majority of their colleagues with respect to sincere interest and enthusiasm in teaching, genuine concern for students, self-study, and continued striving to improve as a teacher (Earls 1981). Earls found that:

- Teachers' personal qualities are developed prior to professional preparation
- Distinctive teachers are respected, not feared by their students
- The positive expectations conveyed by distinctive teachers are reflected in their students' participation and personal behavior
- Distinctive teachers love students
- Authentic-more authentic, less authoritarian over the years
- Continue to change, rather then entrench over time
- Empathy
- Individually
- Openness
- Regard each student as special and unique
- Earned respect as opposed to demanded it

Insights into Excellence: Teachers of the Year

A common trend among teachers of the year in physical education is their emphasis on being an enthusiastic, professional role model. As one teacher of the year (Strategies, Nov-Dec 1989) explained:

> The image we project of our personal self, our enthusiasm for the topic, our knowledge of concepts, and our ability to demonstrate skills combine to create that professional role model which we should strive to perfect. The single concept of role modeling and the image I project to my students dominates my personality and dictates my behavior as a teacher. Pride in myself, in my subject, and in my profession drives me to be the best I can be.
>
> Susan Kogut, National Teacher of the Year

The Elements of Expertise

Expert performance is defined as consistent superior performance on a set of relevant tasks in a specific field of human activity (Bereitner & Scardamalia 1993; Ericsson & Smith 1991). Tan (1997) has described the elements of expertise as follows:

- Extensive knowledge base and domain specificity
- Organize knowledge in a hierarchy
- High level of perceptual capacities
- Experts invest time identifying, defining, and analyzing a problem before searching for a solution

- Automaticity of behavior
- Superior memory
- Superior self-monitoring skills, objectively and honestly assess their shortcomings

To promote expertise, marrying up new teachers with a mentor provides the beginner with an opportunity to observe experienced professionals at work performing the same duties that face the beginner (Bell 1997).

The Science of Teaching

Characteristics of Expert Physical Education Teachers (Manross & Templeton 1997)

- Planning—thorough and complete
- Form a clear, thorough picture of what they are going to do, who they are going to teach, and what equipment they will use
- They look for specific information about their students to gear their lessons towards the students' level of competence
- Make effective and creative use of the teaching environment (facilities, equipment, supplies)
- Greatest difference—experts develop contingency plans
- Use "if this—then that" planning
- Have logical and detailed skill progressions and concepts

Figure 2.3   Expert Teacher

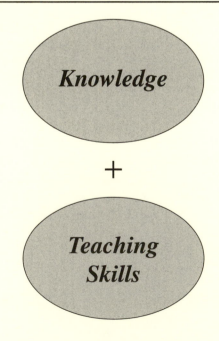

- Recall similar students and search for events and activities that bear on their current class
- Focus on individual student performance
- Intensely focus on individual student learning and performance while keeping the class engaged and on-task (Housner & Griffey 1985)
- Know many ways to present information to learners (Manross et al. 1994)
- Provide a variety of strategies to students who struggle
- Large response repertoires: (Tackle box—bag of tricks)
- Heightened perceptual abilities
- Acutely aware of what is happening
- Develop an early warning system: Detect slight but significant changes in the learning
- Develop automaticity of behavior
- Defined as smooth, effortless, casual, intuitive, and automatic
- Established routines for starting and stopping class, distributing equipment, signals for listening
- Provides specific, creative feedback
- Attain command of subject matter
- Use reflective practices
- Continually analyze their performance soon after the lesson and seek new ways to teach familiar subject matter
- Communicate with other teachers
- Store activities that are particularly successful
- Don't perceive themselves as experts

Nine Points of Effective Teachers

Siedentop (1991) has summarized some key points regarding the practices and behaviors of effective teachers:

1. Ensure that students have ample time and opportunity to practice skills.
2. Set high, yet realistic, expectations which are communicated with clearly defined teacher/student roles.
3. Effective classroom management provides for high amount of student engagement time.
4. Assign meaningful tasks that allow for high success rates.
5. Ensure a brisk pacing and consistent momentum which eliminates student-waiting time.
6. Active teaching: Content is communicated directly with short demonstrations followed by ample guided practice.
7. Active supervision: Supervise practice—do not allow students to move to independent practice too soon.
8. Students are held accountable for completing learning tasks.
9. Effective teachers communicate clearly, are enthusiastic, and maintain a warm classroom environment.

The Data Bank II studies at Columbia University, which focused on outstanding physical programs, revealed a number of interesting findings concerning teachers. Clearly, outstanding teachers were a significant reason for these programs being outstanding. These teachers were thoughtful professionals. Reflection plus experience was a common characteristic of these teachers (Peterson, Allen, & Minotti 1994).

One of the characteristics of teachers in outstanding physical education programs was the relationships they had developed with one another. Positive and supportive relationships among these teachers were very evident (Gay & Ross 1994). These relationships were cultivated by:

Formal Collaboration

- Group planning
- Assist at each other's special events
- Utilization of colleagues as a resource
- Regularly scheduled group meetings

Informal collaboration

- Help out in each other's classes
- Team teaching interactions
- Free exchange of ideas: Informal, spontaneous communications

Summary

Teaching is a complex endeavor. There is no simple prescription to ensure student learning. Each class environment is unique. What appears to be just the right amount of practice time for one class may be too much for another and yet not enough for a third. Class size, students' skill levels, age, and many other things are factors which contribute to the strategies that an effective teacher will use to organize activities and structure the learning environment. Brophy and Good (1986) conclude that "those that teach successfully produce significantly more achievement than those who do not, but doing them successfully demands a blend of knowledge, energy, motivation, and communication and decision-making skills that many teachers, let alone ordinary adults, do not possess."

REFERENCES

Anderson, W. G. (1980). *Analysis of teaching physical education.* St. Louis: C.V. Mosby Company.

Austin, D. A., & Wilhelm, M. (1986). A curriculum development study—school/community collaboration. *Journal of Physical Education, Recreation and Dance. 57* (9), 50–55.

Barrette, G. T. (1977). *A descriptive analysis of teacher behavior in physical education.* Unpublished doctoral dissertation, Teachers College, Columbia University.

Beauchamp, L., Darst, P.W., & Thompson, L.P. (1990). Academic learning time as an indication of quality high school physical education. *Journal of Health, Physical Education, Recreation and Dance. 61*(1).

Beidler, P.G. (1997). What makes a good teacher? In Roth, John K., ed. *Inspiring teaching*. Boston, MA: Anker Publishing Company.

Bell M. (1997). The development of expertise. *Journal of Health, Physical Education, Recreation and Dance. 68* (2), 34–38.

Bereitner, C., & Scardamilia, M. (1993). *Surpassing ourselves*. Chicago: Open Court.

Berliner, D. C. (1994). Expertise: The wonder of exemplary performances. In J. Mangieri, & C. Block (Eds.), *Creating powerful thinking in teachers and students: diverse perspectives* (pp. 161–186). Fort Worth: Harcourt Brace College.

Boyce, B. A. (1989). Goal setting: The ground rules. *Strategies. 3* (2), 22–28.

Brophy, J. (1981). Teacher praise: A functional analysis. *Review of Educational Research. 51*, 5–32.

Brophy, J., & Evertson, C., (1976). *Learning from teaching: A developmental perspective*. Boston: Allyn & Bacon.

Brophy, J., & Good, T. (1986). Teacher Behavior and Student Achievement. In Wittrock, M.C. (1986). *Handbook of Research on Teaching.* 3rd Edition. New York: Macmillan Publishing Company.

Butler, L.F. (1993). *Data Bank II: Case studies of outstanding physical education programs (Case 2).* Unpublished doctoral dissertation. Teachers College, Columbia University.

Butler, L.F. & Mergardt, R. (1994). The Many Forms of Administrative Support. *Journal of Health, Physical Education, Recreation and Dance. 65*, (7) 43–47.

Carre, F.A., Mosher, R., Schutz, R., Thompson, R., Farenholtz, E., & Bullis, L. (1983). *British Columbia assessment of physical education, general report*. Province of British Columbia: The Ministries of Education.

Charles, C.M. (1985). *Building classroom discipline: From models to practice*. New York: Longman, Inc.

Chung, T. B. (1985). *A descriptive study of teaching physical fitness: Time on task in a non-school setting*. Unpublished doctoral dissertation, Teachers College, Columbia University.

Clark, C. M., & Yinger, R. J. (1979). Teacher's thinking. In P.L. Peterson & H.J. Walberg (Eds.), *Research on Teaching*. (pp. 231–263). Berkeley, CA: McCutchan.

Clark, C.M. & Yinger, R.J. (1979). *Three studies of teacher planning* (Research series No. 55). East Lansing, Michigan State University.

Connors, R.D. (1978). *An analysis of teacher thought processes, beliefs, and principles during instruction*. Unpublished doctoral dissertation, University of Alberta, Edmonton, Canada.

Cooke, N., Heron, T., & Heward, W. (1983). *Peer tutoring*. Columbus, OH: Special Press.

Costello, J. (1977). *A descriptive analysis of student behavior in elementary school physical education classes*. Unpublished doctoral dissertation, Teachers College, Columbia University.

Costello, J. & Laubach, S. (1978). Student behavior. In W. G. Anderson and G. Barrette (Eds.), *What's going on in gym. Motor Skills: Theory into practice, Monograph 1,* 11–23.

Cruz, L. M. (1991). *A multi-case study of beginning physical education teachers at the elementary level*. Unpublished doctoral dissertation, Teachers College, Columbia University.

Dauer, V. P. & Pangrazi, R. P. (1989). *Dynamic Physical Education for Elementary School Children*. New York: Macmillan Publishing Co.

Docheff, D. (1990). The feedback sandwich. *Journal of Health, Physical Education, Recreation and Dance*, November/December.

Doolittle, S. A., & Girard, K. T. (1991). A dynamic approach to teaching games in elementary physical education. *Journal of Physical Education, Recreation, and Dance. 62* (4), 57–62.

Doyle, W. (1986). Classroom management and organization. In M. Wittrock (Ed). *Handbook of research on teaching* (3rd ed). (pp. 392–431). New York: McMillan.

Dreyfus, H.L., & Dreyfus, S.E. (1986). Why skills cannot be represented by rules. In N.E. Sharkey (Ed.), *Advances in cognitive science 1* (pp. 313–335).Chichester, England: Horwood.

Earls, N. F. (1981). Distinctive teachers' personal qualities, perceptions of teacher education and the realities of teaching. *Journal of Teaching in Physical Education. 1* (1), 59–70.

Eisner, E. (1983). The art and science of teaching. *Education Leadership. 40* (January), 4–13.

Ericsson, K. A., & Smith. J. (Eds.) (1991). *Toward a general theory of expertise*. Cambridge, MA: Cambridge University Press.

Firestone, W.A. & Pennell, J.R. (1993). Teacher commitment, working conditions, and differential incentive policies. *Review of Educational Research. 63* (4), 484–526.

Fishman, S., & Tobey, C. (1978). Augmented feedback. In W. Anderson, and G. Barrette (Eds), *What's going on in gym. Motor skills: Theory into practice, Monograph 1*, 51–62.

Gage, N.L. (Ed.) (1963). *Handbook of teaching*. American Educational Research Association. Chicago, IL: Rand McNally.

Gallup, G. H. (1984). The 18th Annual Gallup Poll of the Public's Attitude Toward the Public School's. *Phi delta Kappa. 68* (1), 43–59.

Gallup, G. H. (1986). The 16th Annual Gallup Poll of the Public's Attitude Toward the Public School's. *Phi Delta Kappa. 66* (1), 23–28.

Gassner, G. & Sachs, M. (1997). *Comparison of three different types of imagery on performance outcomes in strength-related tasks with collegiate male athletes*. Unpublished doctoral dissertation, Temple University.

Gay, D.A., & Ross, J.R. (1994). Supportive Relationships. *Journal of Health, Physical Education, Recreation and Dance. 65*, (7), 27–30.

Goc-Karp, G. & Zakrajsek, D. B. (1987). Planning for learning—theory into practice? *Journal of Teaching in Physical Education. 6*, 377–392.

Gorden, D. (1978). *Therapeutic metaphors*. Cupertino, CA: Meta.

Gould, D., & Roberts, G. (1982). Modeling and motor skill acquisition. *Quest. 33*, 214–230.

Graham, G., Holt/Hale, S.A., & Parker M. (1987). *Children Moving* (2nd ed.). Mountain View, CA: Mayfield Publishing Company.

Graham, G., Holt/Hale, S.A., & Parker M. (1993). *Children Moving* (3rd ed.). Mountain View, CA: Mayfield Publishing Company.

Graham, K.C. (1996). Running ahead: Enhancing teacher commitment. *Journal of Health, Physical Education, Recreation and Dance. 67*, (1).

Harter, S. (1978). Effectance motivation reconsidered. *Human Development. 21*, 34–64.

Harter, S. (1981). A model of intrinsic mastery motivation in children: Individual differences and developmental change. In W. A. Collins. (Ed.), *Minnesota symposium on child psychology*, Vol. 14 (pp. 215–255). Hillsdale, NJ: Erlbaum.

Highlet, G. (1954). *The Art of Teaching*. New York: Vintage Books.

Housner, L.D., & Griffey, D. (1985). Teacher Cognition: Differences in planning and interactive decision making between experienced and inexperienced teachers. *Research Quarterly for Exercise and Sport. 56*, 44–53.

Imwold, C. H., Johnson, D. J., & Rider, R. A. (1982). The use of evaluation in public school physical education programs. *Journal of Teaching in Physical Education. 2* (1) 13–18.

Jansma, P., French, R., & Horvat, M. A. (1984). Behavioral engineering in physical education. *Journal of Physical Education, Recreation, and Dance. 55* (6), 80–81.

Jensen, E. (1988). *Super-Teaching*. CA: Turning Point

Kneer, M. (1986). A description of physical education instructional theory/practice gap in selected secondary schools. *Journal of Teaching in Physical Education, 5*. 91–96.

Kounin, J. (1970). *Discipline and Group Management in classrooms*. New York: Holt, Rinehart & Winston.

Kounin, J. (1977). *Discipline and Group Management in classrooms*. Melbourne: R. E. Krieger Publishing Company.

Locke, L. & Dodds, P. (1981). Research on pre-service teacher education in the USA. *Artus: Revista de Educacao Fissca e Desportos. 9* (11), 60–67.

Loughrey, T. J. (1975). *Do public school teachers measure—A challenge*. Paper presented at the C.I.C. Symposium on Measurement and Evaluation in Physical Education, Indiana University, Bloomington, IN.

Luke, M. D. (1989). Research on class management and organization: Review with implications for current practice. *Quest. 41*, 55–67.

Mancini, V. H., Cheffers, J. T., & Rich, S. M. (1983). Promoting student involvement in physical education by sharing decisions. *International Journal of Physical Education. 20* (3) 16–23.

Mann, T.R. (1975). The practice of planning: The impact of the elementary school on teacher's curriculum decision making. *Dissertation Abstracts International*, 36/06, 3359A–3360A. (University Microfilms No. 7526968).

Manross, D., Tan, S., Fincher, M., & Schempp, P. (1994). *The influence of subject matter expertise on pedagogical content knowledge in physical education*. Paper presented at the American Educational Research Association annual meeting, New Orleans, LA.

Manross, D., & Templeton, C.L. (1997). Expertise in teaching physical education. *Journal of Health, Physical Education, Recreation and Dance. 68* (3), 29–35.

Marks, M. (1988). A ticket out the door. *Strategies. 1* (2) 17–27.

McLeish, J. (1985). An overall view. In B. Howe & J. Jackson (Eds.). *Teaching effectiveness research* (pp. 68–86). Physical Education Series No. 6. Victoria, B.C.: University of Victoria.

Merriman, E. L. (1976). Considerations identified by elementary teachers as elements of their planning for instructional activities. *Dissertation Abstracts International*, 36/07, 4420A–4421A. (University Microfilms No. 76596).

Morton, P. J. (1989). Contract teaching. *Strategies. 2* (5) 13–16.

Mosston, M. (1966). *Teaching Physical Education: From Command to Discovery.* Columbus, OH: Charles E. Merrill

Mosston, M. (1981). *Teaching physical education* (2nd ed.). Columbus, OH: Merrill.

Mosston, M., & Ashworth, S. (1986). *Teaching Physical Education.* (3rd edition). Columbus, OH: Merrill Publishing Company.

Nichols, B. (1990). *Moving and Learning: The Elementary School Physical Education Experience.* St. Louis: Times Mirror/Mosby College Publishing Co.

Oxendine, J.B. (1970). Emotional arousal and motor performance. *Quest. 13*, 23–30.

Pemberton, C. & McSweigin, P.J. (1989). Goal setting and motivation. *Journal of Physical Education, Recreation, and Dance. 60* (1), 39–41.

Peterson, P. (1979). Direct Instruction Reconsidered. In P. Peterson and H. Walberg, (Eds.), *Research on Teaching: Concepts, Findings, and Implications.* (pp. 57–69) Berkeley, CA: McCutchan.

Peterson, S.C., Allen, V.L., & Minotti, V.L. (1994). Teacher Knowledge and Reflection. *Journal of Health, Physical Education, Recreation and Dance. 65*, (7), 31–37.

Peterson, S. C. (1991). *A multi-case study of instructional sequencing in elementary school physical education.* Unpublished doctoral dissertation, Teachers College, Columbia University.

Philips, D.A. & Carslisle, C. (1983). A comparison of physical education teachers categorized as most and least effective. *Journal of Teaching in Physical Education. 2*, 55–67.

Pieron, M. (1981). Research on teacher change: Effectiveness of teaching a psychomotor task in a microteaching setting. Paper delivered at the American Association of Health, Physical Education, Recreation and Dance Convention, Boston.

Pieron, M., & Graham, G. (1984). Research on physical education teacher effectiveness: The experimental teaching units. *The International Journal of Physical Education, XXI.* (3), 9–14.

Placek, J. (1983). Conceptions of success in teaching: Busy, happy and good? In T. Templin, & J. Olson (Eds.), *Teaching in physical education.* 46–56. Champaign, IL: Human Kinetics.

Placek, J.H. (1984). A multi-case study of teacher planning. *Journal of Teaching in Physical Education. 4*, 39–49.

Quarterman, J. A. (1977). *A descriptive analysis of physical education teaching in the elementary school.* Unpublished doctoral dissertation, Ohio State University.

Reyes, P. (1990). Introduction: What research has to say about commitment, performance, and productivity. In Pedro Reyes (Ed.), *Teachers and their workplace: Commitment, performance, and productivity* (pp. 15–20). Newbury Park, CA: SAGE Publications, Inc.

Rink, J.E. (1985). *Teaching Physical Education for learning.* St. Louis: Times Mirror/Mosby College Publishing Co.

Rosenholtz, S.J. (1989). *Teachers work-place: The social organization of schools.* New York: Longman.

Rosenshine, B. (1979). Content, time and direct instruction. In P. Peterson and H. Walberg, (Eds.), *Research on Teaching: Concepts, Findings, and Implications.* (pp. 28–56) Berkeley, CA: McCutchan.

Rosenshine, B. & Stevens, R. (1986). Teaching functions. In Wittrock, M.C. (1986). *Handbook of Research on Teaching*. 3rd Edition, Macmillan Publishing Company, New York.

Safrit, M. J. (1986). *Introduction to measurement in physical education and exercise science*. St. Louis: Times Mirror/Mosby.

Sander, A.N. (1989). Class management skills. *Strategies. 2* (3) 14–18.

Siedentop, D. (1976). *Developing Teaching Skills in Physical Education*. Boston: Houghton Mifflin.

Siedentop, D., (1983). *Developing Teaching Skills in Physical Education*. (2nd ed.). Mountain View, CA: Mayfield Publishing Company

Siedentop, D., & Eldar, E. (1989). Expertise, experience, and effectiveness. *Journal of Teaching in Physical Education. 8* (3), 254–260.

Siedentop, D., (1991). *Developing Teaching Skills in Physical Education*. California: Mayfield Publishing Company

Siedentop, D., (1995). *Alliance Scholar Lecture*. Paper delivered at the American Association of Health, Physical Education, Recreation and Dance Convention, Portland.

Smith, J.K. (1977). *Teacher planning for instruction* (Report No. 12). Central Midwest Regional Educational laboratory.

Smylie, M.A. (1990). Teacher efficacy at work. In Pedro Reyes (Ed.), *Teachers and their workplace: Commitment, performance, and productivity* (pp. 48–66). Newbury Park, CA: SAGE Publications, Inc.

Stroot, S.A., & Morton, P.J. (1989). Blueprints for Learning. *Journal of Teaching in Physical Education. 8*, 212–222.

Tan, S.K. (1997). The elements of expertise. *Journal of Health, Physical Education, Recreation and Dance. 68* (2), 30–33.

Taylor, P.H. (1970). *How teachers plan their courses*. London: National Foundation for Educational Research in England and Wales.

Tjeerdsma, B.L. (1995). How to motivate students . . . without standing on your head! *Journal of Health, Physical Education, Recreation and Dance. 66*, (5), 36–39.

Tobey, C. (1974). *A descriptive analysis of the occurrence of augmented feedback in physical education classes*. Unpublished doctoral dissertation, Teachers College, Columbia University.

Tyler, R. (1949). *Basic Principles of Curriculum and Instruction*. Chicago: University of Chicago Press.

Veal, M.L. (1988). Pupil assessment perceptions and practices of secondary teachers. *Journal of Teaching in Physical Education. 7*, 327–342.

Wittrock, M.C. (1986). *Handbook of Research on Teaching*. 3rd Edition, Macmillan Publishing Company, New York.

Yinger, R.J. (1977). *A study of teacher planning: Description and a model of pre-active decisionmaking*. (Research Series No. 18). East Lansing: Michigan State University, Institute for Research on Teaching.

Yinger, R.J. (1978). *A study of teacher planning: Description and a model of pre-active decision making* (Research Series No. 18). East Lansing: Michigan State University, Institute for Research on Teaching.

Zahorik, J. A. (1975). Teacher's Planning models. *Educational Leadership. 33*, (2) 134–139.

PART TWO

3

Fitness Walking

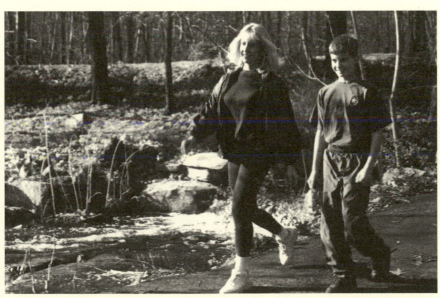

THE NATURE OF FITNESS WALKING

The beauty of walking is that it can be done every day. Fitness walking can be done almost anywhere, and at any time, year around, outdoors, in your neighborhood, in the mall, alone, or with a friend. Walking continues to be the most popular exercise activity in the United States among the 56 sports and fitness activities surveyed by the National Sporting Goods Association. About 67 million men and women are walking regularly. Walking is safe, simple, inexpensive, can be done anywhere, and, due to the low impact nature, is less likely to cause injuries. It's also relaxing and invigorating at the same time, requires little athletic skill, and does not call for a club membership or special equipment. It is fun and natural—good for your mind and self-esteem and benefits most everybody, regardless of age. Unlike many other activities that require specialized equipment or a place to go in order to participate, walking lacks these limiting factors. It is an ideal activity for formal physical education class as part of the curriculum or a community health activity.

EQUIPMENT

Shoes

Good walking shoes are the most important piece of equipment. They provide proper cushioning and stability to the foot and body, which reduces the possibility of injury. Casual shoes with rubber or crepe soles are recommended, with laced shoes offering better support than Velcro slip-ons. Select a lightweight walking shoe with breathable upper materials such as leather or nylon mesh (Figure 3.1). The heel counter should be firm, and the heel should have less cushioning than a traditional running shoe in order to keep the heel closer to the ground for stability. Running shoes often have an elevated heel or one with a wide heel counter. The flatter the shoe, the better. There should be very little height difference between the heel and the toe. The front of the shoe should have good support and flexiblity.

Fit is of the utmost importance with comfort as the key. A good shoe store will fit both feet for length and width with the actual socks that you'll be wearing. It is recommended that you be fitted late in the day because feet will sometime swell during the day and this may affect proper sizing. Shop for shoes right after a long walk when your feet are slightly enlarged. Ensure that the shoe is comfortable, not too tight, and has plenty of room for your toes to move around. There should be approximately 1/2 inch from the big toe to the end of the toe box. Shoes that are too tight or too loose will contribute to blister formation. Spend some time walking around the store in your shoes. Walking or running shoes sometimes run short. Often, your running or walking shoe shoes size will run 1 to 1 1/2 sizes bigger than what you normally wear. Lightly lace your shoes or you may cause foot problems as your feet expand during your walk. Buy an insole with arch support in order to protect yourself from injury if you have a high arch.

Lasts

Many people pronate as they walk. This means that they hit with the heel and then the foot rolls inward with each step. If you roll too far inward, it is known

Figure 3.1   Components of Walking Shoes

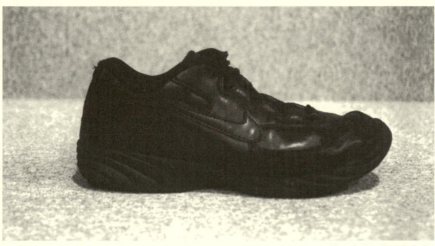

Photo by Matthew G. Butler

as over-pronation. Shoes are made with different lasts in order to prevent this action. If you over-pronate, then straight lasts which have no inward curvature are best. Other lasts are curved, which means they have a noticeable inward curve to enhance the inward rotation. Semi-curved lasts have an area of the sole with construction that prevents the inward rotation to keep the walker from over-pronating. These motion control features are useful in preventing injuries such as tendonitis, bursitis, shin splints, plantar fasciitis, and iliotibial band syndrome. A natural stepping movement is characterized by a slight rolling action with each step. The heel should contact the ground first, and then the foot should roll forward to the toe.

Shoe Life Expectancy

In general, most walking shoes will last for about 500 miles. After this time they will begin to lose their cushioning ability. One strategy is to rotate your shoes by buying a new pair every eight weeks with the same stability, but a different model. This will work different muscles so you will be less likely to have overuse injuries. You can extend the life of your shoe by alternating shoes each time you use them and wearing different shoes for walking, aerobics, and work. In addition, avoid the temptation to buy several pairs at once. Even new shoes that sit around for awhile unused will age due to the drying out of the glue.

Where to Buy Your Shoes

Go to a "technical" shoe store. Most large sporting goods and department stores do not have shoe experts. Talk to friends who walk or run regularly for a reputable source, one where serious runners and walkers buy shoes from experts. These experts will carefully examine your feet and observe your walking gait in order to recommend the best shoe for you. There are many running magazines which will provide lists of good shoe stores. In addition, there are local running clubs which often have their own publications. A good shoe will cost $60–$100. However, spending more than $100 is usually due to style, name brand, or extras that you may not need.

Proper Clothing: Dress for the weather

As with walking shoes, common sense dictates that clothing should be comfortable and lightweight. Clothes that are tight, especially elastic socks, shorts, or garters, have the potential to reduce your circulation. In warm weather, natural cotton fibers are recommended in order facilitate the loss of body heat. In cooler weather, layering is recommended. This layering helps hold heat in, and outer layers can be easily removed as you warm-up. A tremendous amount of body heat is lost through the head, making a hat an essential clothing item on cold days.

Socks

High-quality socks are an important, and often overlooked, item. Great shoes with poor quality socks can lead to foot problems. Many recommend two layers of socks—a thin, soft, inner pair and a regular, padded, outer pair. Many walking experts recommend CoolMax or Thorlo socks. Tube socks should be avoided since they do not fit well over the heel and ankle. One helpful hint is to wash your socks before wearing them to wash out the sizing.

Face Cream

Consider moisturizing cream during the colder months to protect your face, neck, and ears from cold, dry, or windy weather conditions. Almost any name brand will suffice, but it is recommended that you select one which has a sunscreen with a minimum SPF of 15 in order to protect your skin from the damaging effects of the sun.

Reflective Clothing

If you walk in the evening it is essential that you wear clothing with reflective material. There are many types of reflective items available today ranging from reflective vests, which have reflective material sewn in, to reflective belts and arm-bands with built in strobe lights. It is highly recommended that you carry a flashlight in addition to wearing reflective clothing.

Lubricants

Before embarking on your walking adventure, consider using a lubricant on your feet to prevent blisters. There are a number of everyday household items which work well, such as petroleum jelly or talcum powder. There are a number of commercially sold products such as SportSlick and Runners' Lube that are specially designed to help prevent foot blisters. In addition, moleskin or sports tape can be applied if you feel an area of your foot heating up during your walk.

WALKING SKILLS AND TECHNIQUES

Warm-Up

The "warm-up" phase is a very important part of exercising. It consists of a gradual increase in physical activity in order to prepare your body for more strenuous activity. A warm-up period helps prevent muscle soreness and injury and is an essential aspect of exercise program. In the case of fitness walking, the warm-up does not take more than 5-10 minutes and can consist of simply gradually increasing the pace of your walk. By adding some light stretching and strengthening exercises you can complete a solid warm-up in 15 minutes.

Cool-Down

The "cool-down" period is an important time to progressively decrease the level of exercise in order for your body to return to its resting state. Continuous light movements are important in order for your to ensure an adequate return of blood to your heart. This occurs by muscles and one-way valves pumping blood from your legs to your heart. Investing 10 minutes in a gradual cool-down allows your muscles to slowly recover and helps prevent injuries. If time is a concern, then this is also a great opportunity to do some stretching and light strength training.

Getting Started

Although walking is a very natural activity, and it may seem silly to talk about how to walk since we do it every day, there are some important movement patterns one should follow to maximize the fitness aspect. Proper arm movement in particular can enhance and maximize the cardiovascular benefits as well as contribute to proper walking mechanics. In addition, using the proper arm action will enable you to increase your speed. In general, bend your arms at the elbow at an approximate 90-degree angle and keep your hands close to your body. A simple guide is to focus on having your thumbs lightly brush your waist. The arm swing should originate at the shoulders, rather then the elbows.

INSTRUCTIONAL CUES

- Begin your walk slowly and gradually increase speed until you increase your breathing and heart rate.
- Stand tall and keep your eyes and head up.
- Focus your line of sight approximately 10 feet out in front of you—not at your feet.
- Keep your shoulders back and your stomach in.
- Land on your heel—roll forward onto the ball of your foot—and then push off with your toes.
- Take a natural, rhythmical stride.
- Swing your arms freely from the shoulder.
- Breathe deep.

Common Walking Problems and Solutions

Feet that point either in or out can contribute to significant knee problems over time. By keeping your toes pointed forward, as opposed to having your feet pointed either in or out, you can eliminate mechanical problems. In order to assess your walking form, try this movement pattern with a walking partner. Walk down a straight line and have your partner observe your feet to determine the direction that your toes and feet are pointing when you contact the ground. If your feet and toes are pointing either in or out as you walk, you are placing undue pressure on both your ankles and knees. This type of pattern may not cause a problem right away, but may cause injuries over time. Your partner can then provide feedback as you attempt to straighten out your striking pattern.

Improper Stride Length

In order to determine your proper stride length, start in a standing position and lean forward until you begin to naturally fall. Catch yourself with your one leg and look down at your foot. Your foot should be approximately 8 inches in front of your opposite foot. Generally speaking, this is your approximate natural stride length. It will naturally increase as you increase your walking speed. By focusing on short, quick steps you will avoid the tendency to bounce up and down which may create undue stress on your ankle, knee, and hip joints.

Excessive Hip Rotation

Excessive hip rotation is a common problem among walkers. You've probably seen those folks who wiggle as they walk. To eliminate this mechanical problem try this assessment technique. Stand with the side of your body about two inches away from a long wall. Bend your elbow at a 90-degree angle and swing it back and forth from the shoulder trying not to hit the wall with your arm or hand. Once you can do this movement pattern from a stationary position, begin walking forward slowly and continue to swing your arms. The hips will naturally rotate in order to compensate for arms that swing sideways and across your body, so if your arm starts to hit the wall, then that it is a good indication that your hips are over-rotating and wiggling. To remedy this, imagine that there is a wall next to you as you continue your walk.

FOCUS ON FITNESS—TARGET ZONE

As we have learned from the Surgeon General's report on Physical Activity and Health, all forms of activity are beneficial, even in small amounts. However, in order to maximize the health benefits we should follow certain basic principles of exercise. We should gradually build up to the point where we can exercise within our target heart rate zone for 30-60 minutes. To monitor your heart rate, all you need to do is take your pulse. Heart rate monitors are a great investment and simplify this assessment process but certainly are not necessary. If your heart rate is below your target zone during or immediately after exercising, exercise a little harder next time. If you're above your target heart rate, slow down. As a general guide, if you are unable to comfortably carry on a conversation while walking, you need to slow down.

To determine your optimal heart rate, you should reach a training heart rate (THR) which is 65-85% of your maximum heart rate (MHR). The following formula can help you further "personalize" your own training heart rate.

Training Heart Rate (THR) = (65%–85%) Heart Rate Reserve + Resting Heart Rate

Heart Rate Reserve (HRR) = Maximum Heart Rate – Resting Heart Rate

Maximum Heart Rate (MHR) = 220 – Your Age

Resting Heart Rate (RHR) = Your heart rate taken first thing in the morning before getting out of bed or after sitting quietly for 20 minutes

Example: A 40-year-old women has a resting heart rate of 72 beats per minute

THR = (65%) Heart Rate Reserve + Resting Heart Rate

Maximum Heart Rate = 220 – 40 = 180

Heart Rate Reserve = MHR – RHR

Heart Rate Reserve = 180 – 72

Heart Rate Reserve = 108

65% × 108 = 70

70 + 72 = 140

Therefore, this woman's Target Heart Rate is 140 beats per minute.

In addition to this very precise method for determining your training zone, there are other "guides" than can assist you in keeping your heart rate in the training zone.

Music is a powerful motivator and certain styles prompt us to increase or decrease our pace. For example, walking at 3 MPH is equivalent to approximately 120 BPM when listening to marching, rock, mainstream pop, disco, soul, or ragtime. Big band, jazz, square dance, polkas, or Broadway show tunes lend themselves to 4 MPH or 140 BPM. These are simply guides and each individual will respond differently. Hill climbing and interval training will also increase your heart rate significantly with the additional benefit of adding variety to your program.

PROGRESSION—HOW TO START A WALKING PROGRAM

Begin by planning to walk three times a week. Each session should consist of a warm-up period, exercising within your target heart rate zone, and a cool-down period.

You may want to choose the program listed in table 3.1 to get started. Advance according to your goals. Also, consider taking shorter walks five times a week instead of longer walks three times a week.

Beginner

Intensity: Exercise at 50% of your target heart rate. Slow down on hills, at least at first. Walk on level stretches of flat surfaces.

Duration: 10- to 20-minute workouts at the beginning. As you build endurance, you can progress to 30-minute walks. Select a short, flat course.

Frequency: Walk up to three times a week.

Table 3.1
Walking Progression

Week	Distance Walked
1	1/4 mile
2	1/4 mile
3	1/2 mile
4	1/2 mile
5	3/4 mile
6	3/4 mile
7	1.0 mile
8	1.0 mile
9	1.5 miles
10	2.0 miles
11	2.5 miles
12	3.0 miles

Intermediate

Intensity: 70% of your target heart rate.

Duration: Maintain your target heart rate for at least 30 minutes each session.

Frequency: Three to five times a week.

Advanced

Intensity: Start at 75% of your target heart rate; increase your intensity as you build aerobic capacity. Add hills and/or interval training.

Duration: Walk 45 minutes to an hour.

Frequency: Five times per week.

SAMPLE LESSON PLAN

Scope of the Lesson: Introduction to Proper Walking Form

Sequence of the Lesson (45-minute class)

1. Introduce fitness walking as an excellent lifetime activity; increases cardiovascular fitness; muscular endurance; social benefits (5 minutes)
2. Warm-up exercises (5 minutes)
3. Demonstrate proper form and technique—teacher modeling (5 minutes)
4. Review key instructional cues while demonstrating
5. Review student checklist—"instructional cues" (5 minutes)
6. Allow for adequate student practice and individual instruction (20 minutes)
7. Closure—general review of proper walking form/questions (5 minutes)

Major Skill Theme

Proper Walking Form/Technique

Instructional Cues

- Begin your walk slowly, gradually increasing speed until you increase your breathing and heart rate.
- Stand tall and keep your eyes and head up.
- Focus your line of sight approximately 10 feet out in front of you—not at your feet.
- Keep your shoulders back and your stomach in.
- Land on your heel, roll forward onto the ball of your foot, and then push off with your toes.
- Take a natural, rhythmical stride.
- Swing your arms freely from the shoulder.
- Breathe deep.

Suggested learning activities:

1. Teacher models proper walking form and has students provide feedback based on the instructional cues.

2. Students' pair up, observe, and assess their partner's walking form using the checklist as a guide (instructional cues). Students provide individual feedback to one another.

Teaching styles

- Command Style for initial demonstration.
- Individualized Instruction/Practice-Centered (teacher rotates from student to student as students practice proper walking form).
- Reciprocal/Peer assessment utilized by students as they observe one another.

TERMINOLOGY

Board-Lasting: A lightweight board which makes the shoe more rigid. Board-lasted shoes are usually heavier than those having other forms of lasting.

Collar: The opening of the shoe where your foot enters.

Combination-Lasting: Board-lasting is used in the construction of the rear of the shoe, which improves stability, and slip-lasting provides flexibility for the front of the shoe.

Heel Counter: A support component (cup) of the shoe, often made of plastic, which surrounds the heel to assist in overall support and stability.

Insole: The padded surface upon which the foot rests within the shoe. The insole is usually removable for drying purposes, and should be removed if orthotics are used.

Last: The mold around which a shoe is shaped during construction. The last determines the shape and eventual fit of the shoe. Lasts can be straight, semi-curved, or curved; shoes built on different types of lasts provide different types of support and fit options.

Lateral Support: Support provided along the outer portion of the shoe.

Medial Support: Support provided along the inside of the shoe.

Midsole: The material which provides cushioning and is located between the insole and outsole of the shoe.

Outsole: The portion of the shoe that contacts the ground and is designed to provide traction.

Pronation: The normal rolling action of the foot from out to in. This natural action helps absorb the shock. Over-pronation can lead to injury.

Slip-lasting: Construction of a shoe in which the upper, midsole, and outsole are assembled without using a board. Slip-lasting is more flexible and softer than board-lasting or combination-lasting.

Toe Box: The front part of the upper portion that surrounds the toes.

Upper: The portion of the fabric from the sole on up. Usually made of nylon, canvas, or leather.

Wicking: A natural process in which water is moved away from the body due to the nature of a particular fabric. This term is usually used when discussing baselayer fabrics.

SELECTED READINGS

Carlson, B. (1996). *Walking for Health, Fitness and Sport.* Golden, CO: Fulcrum Publishers.

Iknoinan, T. (1995). *Fitness Walking: Technique, Motivation, and 60 Workouts for Walkers.* Champaign, IL: Human Kinetics.

Meyers, C. (1992). *Walking: A Complete Guide to the Complete Exercise.* New York: Random House.

Roberts, S. (1995). *Fitness Walking.* Lincolnwood, IL: Masters Press.

Schlank, K. (1997). *Walking for Fitness & Health.* New York: Sterling Publications.

Smith, K., & Levin, S. (1994). *Kathy Smith's Walkfit for a Better Body.* New York: Warner Books.

The American Heart Association. (1995). *The Healthy Heart Walking Book: The American Heart Association Walking Program.* Indianapolis, IN: Macmillan.

Wood, R.S. (1991). Dayhiker : *Walking for Fitness, Fun and Adventure.* Berkeley, CA: Ten Speed Press.

REFERENCES

Spilner, M. (1998). Walking Fit. *Prevention Magazine.* Emmaus, PA. p. 62.

4

Running

THE NATURE OF RUNNING

Just like fitness walking, the beauty of running is that it can be done almost anywhere, at any time, throughout the year. One of the reasons that running is so popular is its simplicity. Like fitness walking, it requires little athletic skill and does not call for a club membership or special equipment other than sturdy, comfortable shoes. Running is one of the most accessible cardiovascular activities and regardless of where you live, you can almost always find an excellent area for running nearby. Most people can begin by running around the block. The fact that it can be done outdoors, in your neighborhood, is one of the primary reasons that running continues to be one of the most popular exercise activities in the United States. Approximately 22 million men and women are running and jogging regularly. Running is fun and natural, can help promote a positive self-image, and is an excellent way to reduce stress.

Running is also one of the most effective ways to develop cardiovascular fitness. In just 30 minutes a day, 4 days a week, one can achieve an excellent level of aerobic fitness. Few activities burn as many calories as running—making it an excellent part of a sound weight-control program.

Running also provides a great deal of flexibility and variety in training. Variety is one of the most important principles of exercise and promotes adherence. With running, you may choose to run at your own pace, with or without a partner, and at whatever time of day that is convenient for you.

This activity also provides a unique opportunity for the average person on the street to participate in events with national-level athletes, such as large races. However, most people are attracted to events that are low-key, social activities that focus on fun and participation. Running is an ideal activity for all age groups with programs for kids, "masters" programs for older folks, and even family events. In addition, almost every community has a running club.

INSTRUCTIONAL AREA

The beauty of teaching running, and one of the key reasons why it is so popular, is that it can be taught virtually anywhere. Unlike many other activities that require a great deal of specialized equipment or a special place to go in order to participate, running lacks these limiting factors. It is an ideal activity for formal physical education classes, as part of the curriculum, or as a community health activity. It can be taught to high school students on the track or to elementary and middle school students on an athletic field.

As part of the instructional process, the teacher can alert students to the variety of places to run in their community. Road running, running on paths in parks, and cross-country are the most popular. Most people run and race on roads. Here, it is important to run facing traffic so you can see cars coming at you. Many communities have parks with grass or asphalt paths that are designed for walking and running. Running in the woods, on paths, or on golf courses can be exhilarating. Although the running surface is less even in the woods, the soft surface is easier on your joints and helps prevent overuse injuries.

EQUIPMENT

Shoes

Good running shoes are the most important piece of equipment (Figure 4.1). They provide proper cushioning and stability to the foot and body, which reduces the possibility of injury. Running shoes have an elevated heel or one with a wide heel counter as compared to walking shoes.

Fit is of the utmost importance with comfort as the key. A good shoe store will fit both feet for length and width with the actual socks that you'll be wearing. It is recommended that you be fitted late in the day because feet will sometime swell during the day and this may affect proper sizing. Shop for shoes right after a run when your feet are slightly enlarged. Ensure that the shoe is comfortable, not too tight, and has plenty of room for your toes to move around. There should be approximately 1/2 inch from the big toe to the end of the toe box. Running shoe size will run 1 to 1 1/2 sizes bigger than your normal dress shoe size. Shoes that are too tight or too loose will contribute to blister formation. Spend some time walking and jogging around the store in your shoes.

Lasts

Similar to walking, many people pronate as they run. This means that they hit with the heel and then the foot rolls inward with each step. If you roll too far

Figure 4.1   Components of Running Shoes

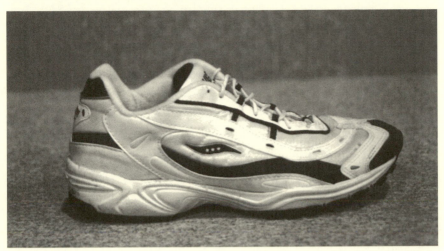

Photo by Matthew G. Butler

inward, it is known as over-pronation. Shoes are made with different lasts in order to prevent this action. If you over-pronate, then straight lasts which have no inward curvature are best. Other lasts are curved, which means they have a notice-able inward curve to enhance the inward rotation. Semi-curved lasts have an area of the sole with construction that prevents the inward rotation to keep the runner from over-pronating. These motion control features are useful in preventing injuries such as tendonitis, bursitis, shin splints, plantar fasciitis, and iliotibial band syndrome. A natural stepping movement is characterized by a slight rolling action with each step. The heel should contact the ground first, and then the foot should roll forward to the toe.

Shoe Life Expectancy

In general, most running shoes will last for about 500 miles. After this time they will begin to lose their cushioning ability. One strategy is to rotate your shoes by buying a new pair every eight weeks with the same stability, but a different model. This will work different muscles so you will be less likely to have overuse injuries. You can extend the life of your shoe by alternating shoes each time you use them and wearing different shoes for running, aerobics, and work. In addi-tion, avoid the temptation to buy several pairs at once because they are on sale. Even new shoes that sit around for awhile unused will age as the glue drys out.

Where to Buy Shoes

Go to a "technical" shoe store. Most large sporting goods and department stores do not have shoe experts. Talk to friends who run regularly for a reputable source, one where serious runners buy shoes from experts. These experts will carefully examine your feet and observe your gait in order to recommend the best shoe for you. There are many running magazines which will provide lists of good shoe stores. In addition, there are local running clubs which often have their own publications. A good shoe will cost $60–$100. However, spending more than $100 is usually due to style, name brand, or extras that you may not need.

Proper Clothing: Dress for the Weather

Clothing should be comfortable and lightweight. Clothes that are tight, especially elastic socks, shorts, or garters, have the potential to reduce your circulation. In warm weather, natural cotton fibers are recommended in order facilitate the loss of body heat. In cooler weather, layering is recommended. This layering helps hold heat in, and outer layers can be easily removed as you warm-up. A tremendous amount of body heat is lost through the head and extremities, making a hat and gloves essential clothing items on cold days. In warmer weather, select a baseball type cap, with a vented mesh top, in order to allow body heat to escape.

Reflective Clothing

If you run in the evening it is essential that you wear clothing with reflective material. There are many types of reflective items available today ranging from reflective vests, which have reflective material sewn in to reflective belts and arm-bands with built in strobe lights. It is highly recommended that you carry a flashlight in addition to wearing reflective clothing.

Socks

High-quality socks are an important, and often overlooked, item. Great shoes with poor quality socks can lead to foot problems. Synthetic fabrics often work better than cotton. Many experts recommend CoolMax or Thorlo socks. Tube socks should be avoided since they do not fit well over the heel and ankle. One helpful hint is to wash your socks before wearing them to wash out the sizing. Many runners prefer socks that are thin, lightweight, and ankle high.

Running Shorts

Loose fitting shorts, with a sidecut, are an excellent choice with most people. Running shorts come with built-in liners, eliminating the need for undergarments.

Undergarments

The Jog Bra is an important consideration for women. It provides extra support and can be worn under a regular T-shirt. If additional support is needed, a second bra can be worn under the jog bra. These items can be purchased in most sporting goods stores.

Outerwear

Nylon tights are a comfortable choice for protecting the legs during cold weather. They do not inhibit your range of motion and help prevent chafing of the legs. Old-fashioned sweats are still an excellent choice for simple, health-related fitness runs.

Face Cream

Consider moisturizing cream during the colder months to protect your face, neck, and ears from cold, dry, or windy weather conditions. Almost any name brand will suffice, but it is recommended that you select one which has a sunscreen with a minimum SPF of 15 in order to protect your skin from the damaging effects of the sun.

Lubricants

Before heading out on your run, consider using a lubricant on your feet to prevent blisters. There are a number of everyday household items which work well, such as petroleum jelly or talcum powder. There are a number of commercially sold products such as SportSlick and Runners' Lube that are specially designed to help prevent foot blisters. In addition, moleskin or sports tape can be applied if you feel an area of your foot heating up during your run. Blisters are caused by friction and this causes fluid to form beneath the skin as a natural defense mechanism.

Here are some preventative measures you can take to avoid blister formation:

- Keep your feet dry.
- Wear insoles.
- Wear acrylic or polyester socks, not cotton.
- Ensure that your shoes fit properly. Shoes that are too small or too big can contribute to the formation of blisters.
- Use a commercial lubricant such as SportSlick or Runners' Lube.
- Use a moleskin covering on areas most likely to blister.

RUNNING SKILLS AND TECHNIQUES

Warm-Up Phase

The warm-up phase is a gradual increase in physical activity that prepares your body for more strenuous exercise. It can be done in 5-10 minutes by gradually increasing the pace of your run. Some light strengthening and flexibility exercises are also recommended during this time period. A warm-up period helps prevent muscle strain and is essential for safe running.

Cool-Down Phase

The cool-down phase involves a gradual decrease in physical activity that facilitates your body's transition back to a resting state. Light physical activity during this phase helps pump blood back up from your legs to your heart. Spending 5-10 minutes gradually slowing your movements allows your muscles to cool off and helps to avoid heart-related problems. This cool-down period is a great opportunity to do light strengthening and flexibility exercises.

INSTRUCTIONAL CUES: RUNNING FORM

- Start off slow
- Run upright, back straight
- Look straight ahead, eyes focused 10 yards in front
- Run in a straight line
- Swing your arms naturally
- Maintain an approximate 90-degree angle at the elbow
- Loosely cup your hands
- Allow your foot to roll forward, from heel to toe, as your shoe contacts the ground

FOCUS ON FITNESS—TARGET ZONE

As we have learned from the Surgeon General's report on Physical Activity and Health, all forms of activity are beneficial, even in small amounts. However, in order to maximize the health benefits we should follow certain basic principles of exercise. We should gradually build up to the point where we can exercise within our target heart rate zone for 30 to 60 minutes. To monitor your heart rate, all you need to do is take your pulse. Heart rate monitors are a great investment and simplify this assessment process but certainly are not necessary. If your heart rate is below your target zone during or immediately after exercising, exercise a little harder next time. If you're above your target heart rate, slow down.

To determine your optimal heart rate, you should reach a training heart rate (THR). This is 65-85% of your maximum heart rate (MHR). The following formula can help you further "personalize" your own training heart rate.

Training Heart Rate (THR) = (65%–85%) Heart Rate Reserve + Resting Heart Rate

Heart Rate Reserve (HRR) = Maximum Heart Rate – Resting Heart Rate

Maximum Heart Rate (MHR) = 220 – Your Age

Resting Heart Rate (RHR) = Your heart rate taken first thing in the morning before getting out of bed or after sitting quietly for 20 minutes

Example: A 40-year-old women has a resting heart rate of 72 beats per minute

THR = (65%) Heart Rate Reserve + Resting Heart Rate

Maximum Heart Rate = 220 – 40 = 180

Heart Rate Reserve = MHR – RHR

Heart Rate Reserve = 180 – 72

Heart Rate Reserve = 108

65% 108 = 70

70 + 72 = 140

Stretching

Stretching is an essential part of an exercise program and especially important for injury prevention in running. It is important that your muscles be warmed up prior to performing flexibility exercises. This can be easily accomplished by jogging lightly or performing light calisthenics for several minutes prior to stretching. Once your muscles are warmed up, stretching will be easier and more effective. You should experience no pain while you stretch. All movements should be slow, gentle, and held for 30-60 seconds. Stretches should be performed in a "static" manner as opposed to a "ballistic" action in which quick, bouncing movements occur. This bouncing movement activates the "stretch reflex" which is the body's natural defense against fast, quick, stretching movements. There are many stretching exercises. Here are a few examples of some common stretches for runners:

Upper-Back Stretch: Stand with feet shoulder-width apart, clasp hands, and raise your arms until they are parallel to the ground. Begin the stretch by reaching forward and rounding (hunching) your upper back. Hold for 30-60 seconds. Repeat.

Back-Saver Hamstring Stretch: Sit with one leg straight and the other bent with the sole of your foot facing the straight leg. Begin the stretch by reaching forward toward your toes with a straight back. Hold for 30-60 seconds, switch legs, and repeat.

Calf and Achilles Tendon Stretch: Stand three feet from a wall (facing the wall). Place your hands on the wall, and begin the stretch by leaning forward with your hips, stretching the calf muscles (keep your heels on the ground). You can vary this exercise by stretching first one leg and then the other. Hold for 30-60 seconds and repeat.

Quadriceps Stretch: Lie down on your right side. Reach back with your left hand and grab your left ankle. Begin the stretch by pulling your left leg back until you feel a gentle stretch on the front of your left thigh. Hold for 30-60 seconds, switch legs, and repeat.

Seated Groin Stretch: Sit on the floor with your back straight. Bend your knees and pull your legs together so the soles of your feet are touching. Your knees will now be pointing outward. Wrap your hands around your feet and lean forward towards your feet. This will stretch the muscles around the groin and hips. Hold for 30-60 seconds. Repeat.

Hip and Back Stretch: Sit with left leg straight, cross your right leg over your left knee and place your left elbow against your right knee. Begin the stretch by turning your trunk (look backward) and pushing your elbow against your knee to facilitate the rotation. Hold for 30-60 seconds, switch legs, and repeat.

At the conclusion of your run, use flexibility exercises as part of your "cool-down" phase.

PROGRESSION: HOW TO START A RUNNING PROGRAM

Begin by planning to jog/walk three times a week. It is important to have an adequate recovery period between runs so begin by having a least one day's rest between sessions. Each session should consist of a warm-up period, exercising within your target heart rate zone, and a cool-down period. A common error among novice runners is to do too much, too soon. Your workload (running time and mileage) should increase gradually. You may want to try the program listed below (based on mileage) as a guide to help you get started. Advance according to your goals, but also listen to your body. Mild muscle soreness is normal at the beginning of a running program. Excessive muscle soreness, however, is often an indicator of over-training.

If you have been performing other cardiovascular activities and are reasonably fit, you can start your running program at what would be week 7 for the beginner. Gradually increase your workload (time or distance) by no more than 5-10% each week.

Table 4.1
Running Progression

Week	Distance Walked
1	1/2 mile
2	1/2 mile
3	3/4 mile
4	3/4 mile
5	1.0 mile
6	1.0 mile
7	1.5 mile
8	1.5 mile
9	1.75 miles
10	1.75 miles
11	2.0 miles
12	2.0 miles

Beginner

Intensity: Exercise at 50% of target heart rate. Avoid hills by selecting level surfaces.

Duration: 10-15 minute jog/walk workouts at the beginning. Gradually progress to 15 minute jogs.

Frequency : Two to three times per week.

Intermediate

Intensity: Exercise at 70% of target heart rate.

Duration: Maintain target heart rate for 20-30 minutes each session.

Frequency : Three to five times per week.

Advanced

Intensity: Exercise at 75-80% of target heart rate; increase intensity as you gradually increase aerobic capacity. Add hills and/or interval training.

Duration: 30-60 minutes.

Frequency: Four to fives times per week.

Running Safety

* Do not use headphones: Headphones eliminate your ability to hear an oncoming car, bike, or other potential hazard.
* Wear reflective material for evening runs.
* Keep emergency identification and/or medical alert information on your person.
* Hydrate: Proper hydration is essential. Even if humidity and temperature are in a comfortable range, vital fluids need to be replaced. Sixty-four ounces of water is required each day before exercise is taken into account. Hydrate before, during, and after your run.
* Let a friend know the run route you plan on taking.
* Don't ignore pain. If you feel pain, stop running immediately.

SAMPLE LESSON PLAN

Scope of the Lesson: Introduction to Three Phases of Exercise for Running

Sequence of the Lesson (45-minute class)

1. Introduce running as an excellent lifetime activity; increases cardiovascular fitness; muscular endurance; social benefits (5 minutes).
2. Review three phases of exercise (5 minutes).

3. Teacher led warm-up phase—teacher modeling (5 minutes).

4. Review heart rate procedures (5 minutes).

5. Training phase: Allow for adequate student practice and individual instruction (15 minutes).

6. Cool down phase.

7. Closure—general review of three phases and student questions (5 minutes).

Major Skill Theme

Three phases of exercise

Instructional Cues

- Three phases of exercise: warm-up, training, and cool-down.
- Warm-up phase is to prepare your body for more strenuous activity.
- Light calisthenics, jogging, followed by stretching exercises are performed during this phase.
- Training phase: Run and gradually attempt to reach your training heart rate. This should take about 5 minutes.
- Check your heart rate several times during your run and adjust your pace as necessary.
- Quick check method: Place index and middle finger on carotid artery (neck). Count heart beat for 10 seconds and multiply by 6 to determine approximate heart rate.
- Cool-down phase: Take 5 minutes to walk slowly and transition to stretching. This allows your body to transition smoothly from high intensity level back to a resting state.

Suggested Learning Activities

1. Brief teacher-led discussion on running as an excellent lifetime cardiovascular activity and review of the three phases of exercise

2. Teacher-led warm-up phase. Teacher models/leads warm-ups and stretches.

3. Review heart rate procedures. Place index and middle finger on carotid artery (neck). Count heart beat for 10 seconds and multiply by 6 to determine approximate heart rate.

4. Training phase: Students jog slowly until they raise reach their training heart rate (65% to start). Maintain this for 5-10 minutes followed by gradual reduction in intensity.

5. Student-led stretches for the cool-down phase.

Teaching Styles

- Command Style for initial demonstration.
- Individualized Instruction/Practice-Centered (teacher rotates from student to student as students practice stretching and learning to determine their heart rate).
- Reciprocal/Peer assessment utilized by students as they observe one another stretch.

TERMINOLOGY

Board-lasting: Construction of a shoe using a lightweight board to aid in the rigidity of the shoe. Board-lasted shoes are generally heavier and stiffer than those having other types of lasting.

Combination-lasting: Construction of a shoe in which board-lasting is used in the rear of the shoe for stability, and slip-lasting is used the front of the shoe for flexibility.

Heel Counter: A support device, usually made of plastic, that surrounds the heel to aid in overall foot support.

Insole: The padded surface upon which the foot rests within the shoe. The insole is usually removable for drying purposes, and should be removed if orthotics are used.

Last: The mold or form around which the shoe is shaped during construction. The last determines the shape and eventual fit of the shoe. Lasts can be straight, semi-curved, or curved; shoes built on different types of lasts provide different types of support and fit options.

Lateral Support: Support provided along the outer side of the shoe.

Medial Support: Support provided along the inside, or arch side, of the shoe.

Midsole: The cushioning materials between the insole and outsole of the shoe.

Outsole: The part of the shoe that comes in constant contact with the ground and is responsible for providing traction.

Pronation: After initial ground contact, the foot is designed to roll inward to disperse shock. Many people roll in too much (over-pronators), causing excessive movement of the foot and lower leg. The reverse of this is a person whose feet don't roll in enough (under-pronators) after ground contact.

Slip-lasting: Construction of a shoe in which the upper, midsole, and outsole are assembled without using a board. Slip-lasting is more flexible and softer than board-lasting or combination-lasting.

Upper: The entire fabric or leather portion of a shoe from the sole up.

Wicking: A process whereby moisture is transported by capillary action. Term most often used in context with baselayer fabrics, but also relevant to other clothing fabrics, sleeping bags, and single-skin tents.

SELECTED READINGS

Benyo, R. (1998). *Running Past 50: A Guide for Getting the Most Out of Your Running in the Second Half-Century of Your Life*. Champaign, IL: Human Kinetics Publishers.

Burfoot, A. (Ed.) (1997). *Runner's World Complete Book of Running: Everything you need to Know to Run for Fun, Fitness, and Competition*. Emmaus, PA: Rodale Press.

Clement, D., & MacNeill, I. (1999). *The Beginning Runner's Handbook*. New York: Sterling Publishing.

Fixx, J. (1977). *The Complete Book of Running*. New York: Random House.

Glover, B. (1996). *The Runner's Handbook*. New York: Penguin USA.

Glover, B. & Lynn Florence, S. (1999). *The Competitive Runner's Handbook*. New York: Penguin USA.

Higdon, H. (1997). *Hal Higdon's How to Train: The Best Programs, Workouts, and Schedules for Runners of All Ages*. Emmaus, PA: Rodale Press.

Lebow, F. (1997). *The New York Road Runners Club Complete Book of Running and fitness*. New York: Random House.

Lyle, M. (1996). *Healthy Runner's Handbook*. Champaign, IL: Human Kinetics Publishers.

Samuelson, J. & Averbuch, G. (1995). *Running for Women*. Emmaus, PA: Rodale Press.

Switzer, K. (1998). *Running and Walking for Women over 40: The Road to Sanity and Vanity*. Torrance, CA: Griffin Trade.

5

Exercising with Equipment: Muscular Fitness Training

THE NATURE OF MUSCULAR FITNESS TRAINING

The Surgeon General's Report on Physical Activity and Health (1996) makes a compelling case for the health benefits that can be accrued from weight training. Muscular Fitness training encompasses a very broad spectrum of activities. Approximately 46 million people engage in activities such as free weights, which include barbells and dumbbells; variable resistance activities such as nautilus equipment; and free body exercises which require no equipment. From a health and wellness perspective, there are many positive changes that occur in the body when a sound muscular fitness training program is followed. There are a number of different types of activities that are related to muscular fitness training:

Resistance Training: A general term that refers to all types of activities and exercises which focus on the development of muscular strength or muscular endurance. There are many modalities that can be used such as free weights, machines, elastic rubber bands, and free body exercises to name just a few.

Weight Training: A generic term that involves any activity which uses free weights or machines. Generally speaking, this activity focuses on strength activities that are conducted for health reasons or for increasing one's strength in order to improve performance in a specific sport. It is not a sport in and of itself like powerlifting or body building.

Powerlifting: A pure strength sport that consists of three events: the squat, the bench press, and the deadlift. Athletes compete in these three events in various categories based on their body weight.

Bodybuilding: A sport in which the primary objective is to develop muscle size for health, aesthetic, and display purposes. Bodybuilders focus on achieving muscular size and symmetry and, like powerlifters, compete in various categories based on their body weight.

INSTRUCTIONAL AREA

Although it is ideal to have access to a facility in which a variety of strength training machines and free weights are available, it is not critical. Most high schools, YMCAs, and community centers will have their own unique set of equipment. Understanding the basic principles of muscular fitness training is the most important requirement. If the basic principles of exercise are known and followed, the type of equipment becomes less of a factor.

EQUIPMENT

There is a great variety of equipment available today and most any type will suffice. The key points are to follow the principles of exercise that are outlined below. In the teaching process, students should be made aware of the different types of equipment. The primary types are as follows:

Constant Resistance Equipment

This type of equipment is characterized by the maintenance of constant resistance (weight) throughout the range of motion. Free weights such as barbells and dumbbells fall into this category.

Variable Resistance Equipment

This type of equipment is characterized by resistance (weight) which changes throughout the range of motion. Nautilus and Cybex equipment are good examples in which the unique shape of the cam inside each machine causes the resistance to change throughout the range of motion.

Multi-Purpose Equipment

Multi-purpose machines have a variety of exercise stations as part of a single unit. Universal gyms are a good example and very common form of this type of equipment. The advantage of this type of equipment is that many exercises can be done in a relatively small area.

Free Body Exercises

Free body exercises require little or no equipment and are comprised of such activities as pushups, pull-ups, and partner resistance exercises to name just a few. You are only limited by your imagination as long as you follow sound principles of strength training.

TYPES OF EXERCISES

Isotonic

A type of resistance training in which you exercise the muscle through the entire range of motion with the resistance (weight) remaining constant. Most types of training equipment falls into this category.

Isokinetic

Isokinetic means same speed. This is a type of resistance training in which the speed of motion is determined by the machine regardless of the amount of force applied. These types of exercises are most common in a therapeutic or rehabilitation setting such as in physical therapy. These machines use either hydraulics or electronics to maintain a constant speed throughout the range of motion.

Isometric

A static type of exercise in which a muscle is exercised at a specific point and there is no joint motion. These types of exercises are very useful if strength is required at a very specific point in a range of motion for a given sport. These exercises tend to significantly elevate blood pressure during the actual execution of the exercise, therefore, people with cardiovascular concerns should check with their physician before embarking on an isometric program.

PHASES OF MUSCULAR CONTRACTIONS

Concentric Phase

During this phase, the muscle is shortening and contracting. For example, during a chin-up, the pulling of the chin up to the bar is the concentric phase. The biceps and Latisimus Dorsi are contracting and shortening.

Eccentric Phase

During this phase of exercise, the muscle is lengthening. The lowering of the body during the chin-up is the eccentric portion. These are also known as "negatives." It is important to focus on both the concentric and eccentric phases of muscular contractions.

MUSCULAR STRENGTH VERSUS MUSCULAR ENDURANCE

Muscular strength is defined as the maximum amount of weight an individual can lift one time. Muscular Endurance refers to the capacity of a muscle group to repetitively contract for an extended period of time. Both aspects of muscular fitness are important, and for purposes of this chapter, we will be focusing on programs which contribute to both of these components of muscular fitness.

PRINCIPLES OF MUSCULAR FITNESS TRAINING

Overload Principle

In order for an increase in strength to occur, a muscle must be overloaded. There must be an increase in the workload of the muscle, either by increasing the resistance or the number of repetitions. Overloading the muscle provides the stimulus for strength gains to take place during the recovery phase. Exercises should be performed until the point of "momentary muscular failure" is reached.

Progressive Resistance

Progression is the systematic increase in workload. This increase in workload may occur by increasing the amount of weight lifted, increasing the number of repetitions, or increasing the number of sets.

Recovery Principle

Once a muscle has been properly stimulated by following the overload principal, it is essential that it be given adequate time to recover. After intense exercise, in which momentary muscular failure is achieved, it is recommended that the muscles involved be allowed to recover for 72-96 hours.

Principle of Specificity

Based upon the goals and objectives of your training program, it is important to provide resistance to the specific muscle groups you wish to improve. This involves a basic working knowledge of which muscles are involved in which exercises.

Balance Principle

It is important that all of the muscles of the body are properly developed and symmetrical. Overworking one muscle group (agonist) and not its opposite counterpart (antagonist) can lead to an imbalance that can lead to poor posture and even injury.

The simplest way to achieve balance is to exercise opposing muscle groups on alternate days. For example, upper body exercises can be done one day and lower body the next day. Another variation of this principle is to work opposing muscle groups on alternate days (agonist—antagonist).

Variety Principle

Performing the same exercises over a long period of time can lead to boredom which will decrease exercise adherence. By adjusting the volume and intensity, varying the types of exercises and using different forms of equipment you can help avoid this problem.

Realism

Being realistic in developing and adhering to your program is one of the most violated principles of exercise. People often attempt to do too much, too soon, and this also contributes to a decline in exercise adherence. One must set aside a realistic amount of time each week and utilize the available equipment and resources wisely.

Regularity

A systematic program is necessary in which there are regularly scheduled training sessions. In general, one workout per week will maintain or slightly increase muscular fitness, and two to three workouts are required for greater gains.

The "FITT" Principle

The "FITT" principle is a summary guide for developing any type of exercise program. The acronym FITT stands for Frequency, Intensity, Time, and Type. In regards to muscular fitness training, the following "FITT Principle" guidelines are recommended:

Frequency: Refers to the number of times per week that you participate in muscular fitness training. Three times per week is recommended with 48-72 hours between workouts.

Intensity: Refers to how hard you train. Greatest gains will be reached by exercising to the point of "momentary muscular failure."

Time: Refers to the number of sets or repetitions. Another time consideration is performing the concentric phase in 2 seconds and the eccentric phase in 4 seconds of each repetition.

Type: Refers to the specific exercises you select based on your goals and objectives. It is important to select the proper exercises for the specific muscle groups that you want to strengthen.

Table 5.1 provides samples of some common types of exercise modalities and the corresponding muscle groups that they work. This is not meant to be all inclusive but serves to alert the teacher to sample exercises, muscle groups, and types of equipment.

Table 5.1
Sample Exercises and Equipment Types

Muscle Group	Free Weights	Nautilus Machines	Universal Machines	Hammer Machines	Free Body Exercises
Gluteus Maximus (Buttocks)	Squats	Leg Press	Leg Press	Leg Press	Squats with partner on back
Quadriceps (Front of Thighs)	Squats	Leg Extension	Leg Press Leg Extension	Leg Extension	Squats with partner on back
Hamstrings (Back of Thighs)	Squats	Seated Leg Curl	Leg Curl	Seated Leg Curl	Squats with partner on back
Calf	Heel Raises		Calf Press		
Chest	Bench Press Incline Press Flys with dumbbells	Bench Press Super Pull Over 10 Degree Chest	Bench Press	Bench Press Incline Press Decline Press	Partner assisted push ups
Latisimus Dorsi (Back)	Bent Over Row	Torso Arm Super Pull Over Compound Row	Lat Pull down	High Row Low Row Behind neck pull down	Lat Pull down with broom handle and partner
Deltoids	Military Press Side Lateral Raises with dumbbells	Lateral Raise Overhead Press	Shoulder Press		Partner assisted push ups
Triceps	French Curl	Multi-tricep Seated Dip	Triceps Extension Dips	Seated Triceps	Partner assisted push ups
Biceps	Curls	Multi-biceps		Seated biceps	Biceps curls with broom handle and partner
Forearms	Wrist Curl		Wrist Curl	Gripper	Wrist curl with broom handle and partner
Abdominal Muscles	Curl ups with light weight on chest	Rotary Torso Abdominal	Leg Raise Station Sit up station		Crunches Curl ups Leg Raises

Table 5.1—*continued*
Sample Exercises and Equipment Types

Muscle Group	*Free Weights*	*Nautilus Machines*	*Universal Machines*	*Hammer Machines*	*Free Body Exercises*
Lower Back Muscles	Good Morning (back extensions)	Lower back	Back extension		Back extension
Neck		Four Way neck			Partner resistance neck extension and flexion

SAMPLE EXERCISES USING FREE WEIGHTS (SAFETY SPOTTER REQUIRED)

For all exercises, perform the concentric phase (positive) in 2 seconds and the eccentric phase (negative) in 4 seconds. This eliminates momentum and optimizes each repetition.

Name of Exercise: Squats

Muscle Groups: Gluteus Maximus, Quadriceps, Hamstrings

Starting Position: Place feet slightly more than shoulder width apart. Place bar on the muscular portion of your shoulders behind neck (placing a towel under the bar will help cushion and protect your shoulders).

Proper Execution: Lower body by bending at the knees until you are sitting in an imaginary chair. Return to the starting position. Keep the back straight and the head up during each repetition.

Instructional Cues: Back straight, head up, Bend knees to 90-degrees.

Safety Spotter: Two spotters stand on each side of the bar assisting as necessary.

Name of Exercise: Heel Raise

Muscle Group: Calf

Starting Position: Stand with feet slightly more than shoulder width apart. Place bar on shoulders behind neck.

Proper Execution: Raise heels off the ground as high as possible by pushing up with the balls of your feet. Hold this elevated position for one second before returning to the starting position.

Safety Spotter: Spotter stands behind the performer and grasps the bar lightly until assistance is required.

Name of Exercise: Bench Press

Muscle Group: Chest, Deltoids, Triceps

Starting Position: Back flat on bench and feet flat on ground. Grip the bar with hands slightly more than shoulder width apart.

Proper Execution: Lower the bar to your chest in 4 seconds, raise bar until elbows are fully extended in 2 seconds.

Safety Spotter: Spotter stands over the performer, near the head, and grasps the bar lightly until assistance is required.

Name of Exercise: Incline Press

Muscle Group: Upper Chest, Deltoids, Triceps

Starting Position: Back flat on bench and feet flat on ground. Grip the bar with hands slightly more than shoulder width part.

Proper Execution: Same execution as the bench press except the bench is raised so that the upper body is at a 45-degree angle.

Safety Spotter: Spotter stands over the performer, near the head, and grasps the bar lightly until assistance is required.

Name of Exercise: Dumbbell Flys

Muscle Group: Chest

Starting Position: Back flat on bench with one dumbbell in each hand. Start with the arms extended over your chest.

Proper Execution: Bend elbows slightly and lower the dumbbells laterally until you feel a slight stretch in your chest. Return to the starting position.

Safety Spotter: Spotter stands over the performer, near the head, and grasps the dumbbells lightly until assistance is required.

Name of Exercise: Bent-over Row with Dumbbell

Muscle Group: Latisimus Dorsi and Biceps

Starting Position: Kneel on a bench as shown in (Figure 5.1). Bend over at the waist until your chest is parallel to the ground.

Proper Execution: Pull the dumbbell straight upward by lifting your elbow as high as possible, hold for 1 second, and return to the starting position in 4 seconds.

Name of Exercise: Overhead Press

Muscle Group: Deltoids

Figure 5.1   Bent Over Row

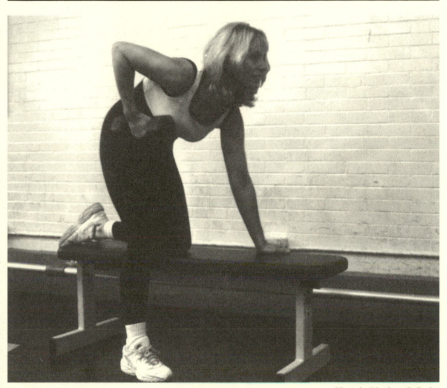

Photo by Matthew G. Butler

Starting Position: Sit on bench with feet flat on the ground and back straight. Place barbell in front of your shoulders with a shoulder-width grip.

Proper Execution: Raise the bar in 2 seconds until elbows are straight, hold for 1 second, and return to the starting position in 4 seconds.

Safety Spotter: Spotter stands behind the performer and grasps the bar lightly until assistance is required.

Name of Exercise: Side-lateral Raise

Muscle Group: Deltoids

Starting Position: Stand with feet slightly more than shoulder width apart. Grasp dumbbells and place at your side. Bend elbows slightly.

Proper Execution: Raise arms laterally, with slightly bent elbows, until they are parallel to the ground. Hold this position momentarily and then return to the starting position.

Safety Spotter: Spotter stands behind the performer and grasps the arms lightly until assistance is required.

Name of Exercise: French Curl

Muscle Group: Triceps

Starting Position: Back flat on bench and feet flat on ground. Grip the bar with a very narrow grip.

Proper Execution: Keep your elbows stationary and lower the bar to your forehead in 4 seconds, raise bar until elbows are fully extended in 2 seconds.

Safety Spotter: Spotter stands over the performer, near the head, and grasps the bar lightly until assistance is required.

Name of Exercise: Biceps Curl with Dumbbells

Muscle Group: Biceps

Starting Position: Stand with feet slightly more than shoulder width apart.

Proper Execution: Keep your elbows stationary and curl the dumbbell upward in 2 seconds. Lower to start position in 4 seconds.

Safety Spotter: Spotter stands in front of the performer and grasps the dumbbells lightly until assistance is required.

Figure 5.2   Biceps Curl

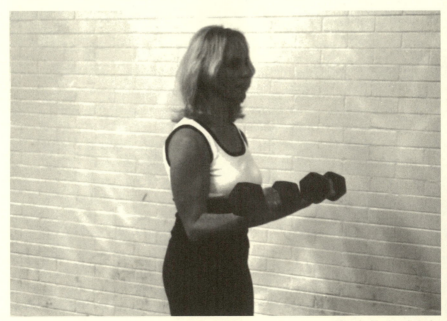

Photo by Matthew G. Butler

Name of Exercise: Wrist curl

Muscle Group: Forearms

Starting Position: Sit on bench with feet flat on ground. Place your elbows on knees and grasp the barbell approximately shoulder width apart.

Proper Execution: Curl bar upward using your wrist and forearms. Hold momentarily and lower to the starting position. As you return to the start position allow the bar to roll down your hands to your fingers.

Safety Spotter: Spotter stands in front of the performer and grasps the bar lightly until assistance is required.

SAMPLE EXERCISES USING MACHINES

There are a great variety of exercise machines available today on the market. They are all different but often move in similar patterns. Often times, schools or community centers have several types available. Follow the instructions carefully regarding the proper way to use each particular make. The exercises provided here can be done in a similar manner on a variety of exercise machines such as Nautilus, Universal, and Hammer Strength equipment.

Name of Exercise: Leg Press

Muscle Groups: Gluteus Maximus and Quadriceps

Starting Position: Adjust the bench until knees are bent at 90-degrees.

Proper Execution: Press legs forward by extending the knees in 2 seconds. Pause momentarily and return to the starting position in 4 seconds.

Name of Exercise: Leg Extension

Muscle Groups: Quadriceps

Starting Position: Sit on bench and grasp handles with hands.

Proper Execution: Extend the legs upward in 2 seconds and hold momentarily. Return to the starting position in 4 seconds.

Name of Exercise: Leg Curl

Muscle Groups: Hamstring

Starting Position: Sit or lie on bench depending on the model. Grasp handles with hands.

Proper Execution: Curl the legs upward in 2 seconds and hold momentarily. Return to the starting position in 4 seconds.

Name of Exercise: Bench Press

Muscle Groups: Chest

Starting Position: Back flat on bench and feet flat on ground. Grip the bar with hands slightly more than shoulder width part.

Proper Execution: Raise bar until elbows are fully extended in 2 seconds. Lower the bar to your chest in 4 seconds.

Name of Exercise: Lat Pull Down

Muscle Groups: Latisimus Dorsi and Biceps

Starting Position: Sit on bench and grasp bar/handle with arms fully extended.

Proper Execution: Pull the bar/handle to your chest in 2 seconds, hold for one second, and return to the starting position in 4 seconds.

Name of Exercise: Overhead Press (Shoulder Press)

Muscle Groups: Deltoid and Triceps

Starting Position: Sit on bench with feet flat on the ground and back straight. Grasp the bar/handle with hands approximately shoulder width apart.

Proper Execution: Raise the bar in 2 seconds until elbows are straight, hold for one second, and return to the starting position in 4 seconds.

Name of Exercise: Triceps Extension

Muscle Groups: Triceps

Starting Position: Sit on bench or stand, depending on model. Grasp bar/handle with a narrow grip.

Proper Execution: Keep elbows stationary and extend arms until fully extended. Hold momentarily and return to the starting position.

Name of Exercise: Biceps Curl

Muscle Groups: Biceps

Starting Position: Sit on bench or stand, depending on model. Grasp bar/handle with a narrow grip.

Proper Execution: Keep your elbows stationary and curl the bar upwards in 2 seconds. Pause momentarily and lower to start position in 4 seconds.

Figure 5.3   Lat Pull Down

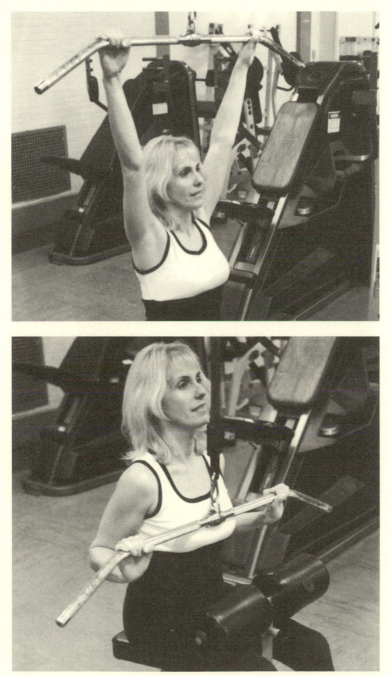

Photos by Matthew G. Butler

Figure 5.4   Overhead Press

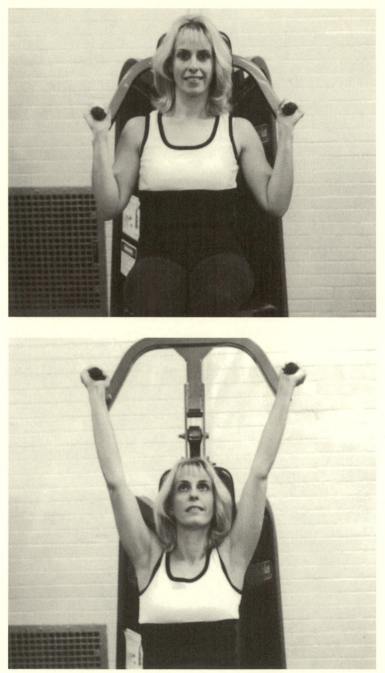

Photos by Matthew G. Butler

Name of Exercise: Leg Raise Station

Muscle Groups: Hip Flexors

Starting Position: Hang from bar.

Proper Execution: Raise legs either straight (advanced) or draw knees to chest in 2 seconds. Hold momentarily, and return to the starting position in 4 seconds.

SAMPLE OF FREE BODY EXERCISES

These exercises require little or no equipment and should be done with a partner who provides the resistance.

Name of Exercise: Squats

Muscle Groups: Gluteus Maximus, Quadriceps, Hamstrings

Starting Position: Select a partner who is of similar size and strength. Performer places feet slightly more than shoulder width apart. Partner piggybacks on performer with hands wrapped around performer's upper body and performer grasps partner's legs.

Proper Execution: Lower body by bending at the knees until you are sitting in an imaginary chair. Return to the starting position. Keep the back straight and the head up during each repetition.

Name of Exercise: Partner-assisted Push-ups

Muscle Groups: Chest, Deltoids, Triceps

Starting Position: Performer assumes a front leaning rest position (push-up) with the partner standing and straddling the back of the performer. Partner places hands on the performer's shoulder blades.

Proper Execution: The partner provides the resistance and should apply enough force so that the performer reaches momentary muscular failure in 8-12 repetitions.

Performer slowly lowers chest towards the ground in 6-8 seconds with the partner providing moderate resistance by pushing on the performer's back. Performer then pushes up in 2-4 seconds with partner again providing moderate resistance.

Name of Exercise: Curl-ups

Muscle Group: Abdominal

Starting Position: Performer lies on back with knees bent at 90-degrees, feet flat, and hands at their side with palms down. Partner kneels behind them and places hands on the front of each shoulder.

Proper Execution: The performer curls up until their shoulder blades are off the ground. The partner providing light resistance with their hands on the performer's shoulder. The partner then gently pulls the performer back to the ground in 4 seconds as the performer resists this movement.

Figure 5.5   Curl Ups

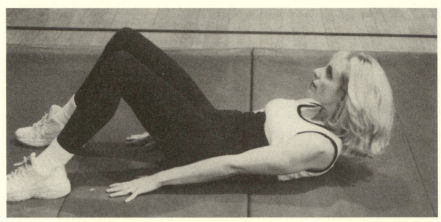

Photo by Matthew G. Butler

The following exercises utilize an inexpensive, three-foot-long wooden dowel, which is approximately one inch in diameter and available in most lumber yards. The partner provides an appropriate amount of resistance on both the positive phase (concentric) and negative phase (eccentric) to ensure that the performer reaches momentary muscular failure in 8-12 repetitions. It is important that both the partner's and the performer's hands are directly next to (touching) one another to eliminate the possibility of the dowel breaking.

Name of Exercise: Lat Pull Down

Muscle Groups: Latisimus Dorsi

Starting Position: Performer sits on the ground with legs crossed, arms extended overhead with dowel in hand. Partner stands behind the performer, places the side of their knee in the performers back for stability, and grasps the dowel.

Proper Execution: Performer pulls the dowel down behind their back in 2 seconds with the partner providing resistance. Partner then pulls up on the dowel causing the performers arms to return to the start position in 4 seconds. The performer resists this movement.

Name of Exercise: Seated Press (Shoulder Press)

Muscle Groups: Deltoids, Triceps

Starting Position: Performer sits on the ground with legs crossed, arms extended overhead with dowel in hand. Partner stands behind the performer, places the side of their knee in the performers back for stability, and grasps the dowel.

Proper Execution: Partner pushes the dowel down behind the performer's back in 2 seconds with the performer providing resistance. Performer then pushes up on the dowel returning to the start position in 4 seconds. The partner provides resistance.

Name of Exercise: Biceps Curl

Muscle Group: Biceps

Starting Position: Performer stands with feet slightly more than shoulder width apart. Grasp the dowel with a shoulder width grip and bend knees slightly. Partner stands directly in front of the performer in a stride position grasping the dowel.

Proper Execution: Performer keeps their elbows stationary and curls the bar upwards in 2 seconds with the partner providing resistance. The partner then pushes downward on the dowel returning it to the starting position. The performer resists this 4-second movement.

PROGRESSION: HOW TO START A MUSCULAR FITNESS PROGRAM

The first step is to identify your goals and objectives. Your programs will vary depending on whether you are interested in developing muscular strength, muscular endurance, or a combination of both. If your primary interest is in developing health-related fitness, then you would focus a program which helps develop both components. A recommended program would include performing 2-3 sets of 8-12 repetitions three times per week. If your goal is to develop muscular strength then, 2-3 sets of 6-8 repetitions should be performed. For muscular endurance, performing 3-5 sets of 15-20 repetitions is recommended.

Beginners should first focus on learning proper form and techniques. A common problem with beginners is attempting to lift too much too soon. For those who are participating in muscular fitness training for the first time, it is recommended that you begin with 1 set of 8-12 repetitions for the first two weeks. Improper technique and too much weight can not only lead to unnecessary soreness and less adherence, but also to injury. Beginners should emphasize proper form, not weight, especially with free weights. Lifting free weights is a skill, and a beginner must learn to balance and coordinate the muscular movements, which takes a number of practice sessions.

SAMPLE LESSON PLAN

Scope of the Lesson: Introduction Free Body Exercises

Sequence of the Lesson

1. Introduce free body exercises as an excellent way to develop muscular fitness. The main advantage of this type of exercise is that little or no equipment is required.
2. Demonstrate proper form and technique in executing six free body exercises (teacher models with a student).
3. Review key instructional cues while demonstrating.

4. Review student checklist with students.

5. Allow for adequate student practice and individual instruction.

6. Closure—general review of proper form and technique/answer questions.

Major Skill Theme

Variety of Free Body Exercises

Instructional Cues

- Squats
  - Back Straight
  - Look Up
  - Bend Knees to 90-degrees
- Partner-assisted push-ups
  - Back Straight
  - Down in 8 seconds, Up in 4 seconds
  - Partner places hands on your shoulder blades
- Lat Pull Down
  - Sit with legs crossed
  - Partner is behind you with side of knee in your back
- Biceps Curl
  - Partner stands in front, facing you
  - Stand with legs shoulder width apart
  - Curl up in 2 seconds, down in 4 seconds

Safety Cues

- Proper Warm-up
- Focus on Proper Form and Technique
- Begin with light weights or resistance
- Breathe properly: Do not hold your breath. Exhale on concentric phase, Inhale on eccentric phase.
- Maintain a safe distance from other lifters
- Don't drop equipment/weights
- Utilize safety spotters
- Use collars on barbells

Suggested Learning Activities

1. Teacher models proper form in demonstrating free body exercises with a student volunteer. Teacher reviews instructional cues for each exercise while demonstrating. Two volunteer students model one of the exercises. Students provide feedback on the demonstration based on the instructional cues.

2. Utilize learning center format (stations). Have several stations for each exercise and have students rotate through the stations. Student's pair up, spot, and assess one another's form using the instructional cues checklist. Students provide individual feedback to one another.

Teaching Styles

- Command Style for initial demonstration
- Individualized Instruction/Practice Centered (instructor rotates from student to student as students practice proper form at each exercise station.
- Reciprocal/Peer assessment utilized by students as they observe one another at each station.

TERMINOLOGY

Atrophy: A decrease in the size of the muscle cells.

Bodybuilding: A sport or activity in which the primary objective is to develop the size of the skeletal muscles. Bodybuilders focus on other areas as well, such as developing all of the muscles proportionally (symmetrically), minimizing body fat and increasing their strength.

Circuit Training: Performing a number of exercises in continuously and in succession in order to enhance muscular and cardiovascular endurance.

Concentric: This is the portion of a muscular contraction in which the muscle shortens.

Constant resistance: A type of muscular fitness exercise in which the workload (weight) remains the same throughout the range of motion.

Eccentric: This is the portion of a muscular contraction in which the muscle lengthens. This is also known as the negative portion.

Free body exercises (No Equipment): Free body exercises require little or no equipment and are comprised of such activities as pushups, pull-ups, sit-ups, and the many variety of abdominal variations.

Free-weights: Barbells and dumbbells

Hypertrophy: An increase in the size of muscle cells.

Isokinetic: A type of resistance in which the speed of motion is determined by the machine.

Isometric: A type of resistance in which there is no joint motion.

Isotonic: A type of resistance training in which the resistance remains the same throughout the range of motion.

One repetition maximum. (Also known as 1 RM.): The maximum amount of weight a person can lift one time.

Powerlifting: A sport that consists of three events: squat, bench press, and deadlift.

Resistance: The workload or amount of weight that is used when exercising.

Resistance Training: Resistance training is a broader term than weight training. Weights, machines, rubber strands and any number of other devices that resist the movement of the exerciser can supply this resistance.

Set: The number of repetitions performed in an exercise.

Variable Resistance Equipment: This type of equipment is characterized by resistance, which changes throughout the range of motion.

Weight Training: Weight training refers to any activity, which involves the use of weights.

SELECTED READINGS

Baechle, T. & Earle, R. (1994). *Fitness Weight Training*. Champaign, IL: Human Kinetics.

Baechle, T. & Groves, B. (1998). *Weight Training: Steps to Success*. Champaign, IL: Human Kinetics.

Bompa, T. & Cornacchia, L. (1998). *Serious Strength Training*. Champaign, IL: Human Kinetics.

Brzyki, M. (1995). *A Practical Approach to Strength Training*. Lincolnwood, IL: Masters Press.

Fahey, T. (1996). *Basic Weight Training for Men and Women*. Mountain View, CA: Mayfield Publishing Company.

Karony, S. & Ranken, A. (1998). *Body Shaping with Free Weights: Easy Routines for Your Home Workout*. New York: Sterling Publications.

Karony, S. (1993). *Workouts with Weights: Simple Routines You Can Do at Home*. New York: Sterling Publications.

Kennedy, R. (1998). *Weight Training Basics*. New York: Sterling Publications.

Kraemer, W. & Fleck, S. (1992). *Strength Training for Young Athletes*. Champaign, IL: Human Kinetics.

Roberts, S. (1994). *Strength and Weight Training for Young Athletes*. Chicago, IL: NTC Contemporary Publishing.

Westcott, W. (1996). *Building Strength and Stamina: New Nautilus Training for Total Fitness*. Champaign, IL: Human Kinetics.

6

In-Line Skating

THE NATURE OF IN-LINE SKATING

In-line skating is one of the fastest growing sports in the United States. The Sporting Goods Manufacturers Association (SGMA) estimates that participation in this activity has grown over 800% in the last eight years. Approximately 29 million people in the United States participate in in-line skating which ranks it 11th in participation out of 66 sports in the SGMA survey. A similar participation trend was identified in the National Sporting Goods Association (NSGA) annual survey of sports participation. This survey found that 26.6 million Americans actively participated in in-line skating in 1997, which was a 4.1% increase from the previous year and a 739% increase from 1990.

There are many reasons for this sport's increased popularity. It is a fun and exciting activity with a relatively low start up cost. It is easily accessible in that you can skate just about anywhere, and finally, skating causes significantly less shock to the knees, hips, and lower back than running. It has attracted many young people who enjoy the excitement of aggressive skating, leisurely skating, or in-line hockey.

INSTRUCTIONAL AREA

Any flat, non-congested area will suffice for in-line skating. In school or college settings, smooth, open, asphalt parking areas that are free from traffic are ideal. The primary concern is to have a traffic-free area so that beginners feel safe, especially when their confidence and control are being developed.

EQUIPMENT

Proper equipment for in-line skating includes quality skates that are properly maintained and protective equipment.

Protective equipment is essential for in-line skaters. Head injuries, in particular, can be life threatening, making a safety helmet the most important piece of protective equipment. From a teaching perspective, wearing protective equipment also contributes to making students' more relaxed and increases their confidence, making learning to skate more enjoyable.

Helmet—This is the most important piece of safety equipment. Helmets should be ASTM, SNELL, or ANSI rated or approved.

Knee Protection—Knee pads help protect the knees from contusions and abrasions. By landing on the knees first during a fall, a skater can help dissipate the landing forces. Ensure that kneepads are firmly secured around the leg with straps.

Elbow Protection—Elbow pads help protect the elbows from contusions and abrasions.

Wrist Protection—When losing control or balance, which is inevitable in the learning process, in-line skaters should be taught to fall forward. Proper wrist protection will prompt sliding which also helps dissipate landing forces.

Skates

Just like walking and running shoes, the most important part of selecting a pair of skates is ensuring a proper fit. Because everyone's feet are different, it is important to spend time on this portion of the selection process. This will help make learning to skate much more enjoyable for students because it will eliminate future blisters, chaffing, and movement of the foot inside the skate. The skate is made of a polyurethane shell which has a liner, and an understructure which contains the wheels, spacers, bearings, and brake. There are many different variations of in-line skates on the market today. Some have thin liners while others have very thick, comfortable liners, and there are even custom inserts available. The liners that lace-up tend to offer better support and often fit better than the stitched type.

Just as with walking and running shoes, many people pronate as they skate. A heel wedge can be of great assistance in correcting this problem, however, a custom insole may be required. To help tailor the fit to the nuances of your feet, pads can be used. A tongue pad can prevent forward and backward movement of your foot in the skate. By placing a pad under your foot, you can help push the foot down if there is upward and downward movement; this helps customize the fit. Pads can also be used just outside the liner if the skate is slightly wide as well as in any area of the foot that becomes sensitive.

There are many different types of in-line skates available today. This includes recreational skates, hockey skates, speed skates, and the aggressive style. The recreational version is an ideal choice for introducing students to the sport. They are lighter than other types and have large, soft wheels. Speed skates are also light in weight but have an extra wheel. Hockey and aggressive skates are more durable in nature.

To maximize your enjoyment and safety while skating, teachers should ensure that their students follow these simple steps:

- Wear protective equipment
- Rotate the wheels
- Clean the bearings
- Check the spacers
- Inspect the brake pads for wear (look for the wear line)
- Ensure the brake is firmly attached
- Adjust the position of the brakes

Selecting Skating Components

When selecting new wheels for your skates, ensure you have the proper diameter (size), durometer (hardness), and profile (shape).

Talk to a knowledgeable salesperson regarding bearing selection and inquire about the following key factors:

- Serviceability
- ABEC Rating (precision)
- Lubrication (speed/maintenance/protection)
- Materials (rings/retainers/shields)
- Internal Geometry (shallow vs. deep groove)

SKILLS AND TECHNIQUES

Learning to Stop

From a safety perspective, learning how to stop is clearly an essential skill and should be taught first. The starting position for teaching this skill consists of positioning your skates a few inches apart (almost touching) and parallel to one another. Face forward with your knees slightly bent. This lowers your center of gravity, thereby improving your balance and stability. Bending your knees also makes it easier to stand up straighter as opposed to leaning forward. In addition, looking forward, not down, will help you maintain a straight back.

Roll your braking skate forward keeping the toe down. When you slide your braking foot forward, make sure it goes straight, not out to the side. Try to get your feet lined up in a straight line as if your are skating on a two-by-four. Wait until your braking foot is well in front of your other foot (preferably at least 6 inches) before lifting your toe. Bending your knees will help facilitate this action. Lifting the toe early will engage the brake too soon. Keep your back fairly straight and lower your center of gravity. If your skates have the ABT brake this step may not be necessary because the ABT should engage as you slide your braking foot forward. Your braking foot should now be approximately 6 inches in front of the toe of your other foot. Keep most of your weight on your braking skate with your center of gravity just behind the braking skate.

Striding

Skating is a rhythmic movement which consists of alternately stroking and gliding. This should be done slowly at first with the weight centered over the gliding skate. Avoid the tendency to use short, rapid strokes.

Summary Checklist

- Wear your protective equipment
- Develop your skating skills, especially stopping and turning
- Maintain your skating equipment
- Follow traffic laws and regulations and avoid traffic when possible
- Skate within your skill limits and always maintain control
- Be alert to road hazards such as oil on road, water, and sand
- Pass on the left
- Yield to walkers

International In-Line Skating Association's Skate Buyers Checklist

Check the type of skating that best reflects your interests.

- Hockey
- Speed
- Freestyle
- Recreational
- Fitness
- Aggressive

What is your budget?

- Under $100
- $100 to $150
- $150 to $200
- $200 to $250
- Over $250

What kind of wheels?

- More speed, less control
- More control, less speed

- Soft, for use on irregular surfaces
- Hard, for use on smooth surfaces
- Specialty (hockey, speed, figure, aggressive)
- Bearings, ABEC rated

What kind of brakes?

- Standard in-line skate brake
- Special braking system

What kind of boot?

- Plastic composition
- Soft boot composition
- Buckle closure system
- Lace closure system
- Lace/buckle combo
- High tech material in liner
- Orthotic footbed
- Specialty boot (hockey, speed, figure, aggressive)

What kind of frame?

- Movable frame
- Rockerable frame
- Standard fixed-frame
- Accepts different sizes of wheels
- Specialty frame (hockey, speed, figure, aggressive)

Assess your future needs

- Buy skates that you can modify as you improve
- Plan to replace skates if you improve

The gear you will buy

- Properly fitted helmet
- Wrist guards, knee and elbow pads

Skate lessons you will take

- Beginner; moving and stopping
- Lesson program or skill-building series

FOCUS ON FITNESS

In-line skating can produce cardiovascular benefits similar to walking and running. In order to maximize the training effects, skaters can utilize a more rapid, continuous skating stroke and minimize the gliding portion. This requires greater control and should only be done in open areas free of traffic and other hazards. The training heart rate formula can be utilized as described in the running chapter. Another way to increase the training effect is to skate uphill. This significantly increases the workload which will raise your heart rate and improve the muscular endurance of the lower body muscles.

Beginner

Intensity: Exercise at 60% of your Training Heart Rate.

Duration: 10-15 minutes in an open area such as an empty parking lot—slow skating.

Frequency: Two to three times per week.

Intermediate

Intensity: Exercise at 70% of target heart rate.

Duration: Maintain target heart rate for 20-30 minutes each session.

Frequency: Three to five times per week.

Advanced

Intensity: Exercise at 75-80% of target heart rate; increase intensity as you gradually increase aerobic capacity. Add hills.

Duration: 30-60 minutes.

Frequency: Four to fives times per week.

Stretches for In-Line Skaters

Back-Saver Hamstring Stretch: Sit with one leg straight and the other bent with the sole of your foot facing the straight leg. Begin the stretch by reaching forward toward your toes with a straight back. Hold for 30-60 seconds, switch legs, and repeat.

Calf and Achilles Tendon Stretch: Stand three feet from a wall (facing the wall). Place your hands on the wall, and begin the stretch by leaning forward with your hips, stretching the calf muscles (keep your heels on the ground). You can vary this exercise by first stretching one leg and then the other. Hold for 30-60 seconds and repeat.

Figure 6.1   Backsaver Hamstring Stretch

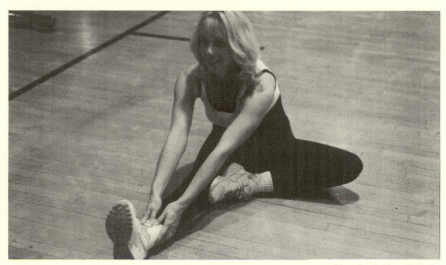

Photo by Matthew G. Butler

Quadriceps Stretch: Lie down on your right side. Reach back with your left hand and grab your left ankle. Begin the stretch by pulling your left leg back until you feel a gentle stretch on the front of your left thigh. Hold for 30-60 seconds, switch legs, and repeat.

Seated Groin Stretch: Sit on the floor with your back straight. Bend your knees and pull your legs together so the soles of your feet are touching. Your knees will now be pointing outward. Wrap your hands around your feet and lean forward towards your feet. This will stretch the muscles around the groin and hips. Hold for 30-60 seconds. Repeat.

Hip and Back Stretch: Sit with left leg straight, cross your right leg over your left knee and place your left elbow against your right knee. Begin the stretch by turning your trunk (look backward) and pushing your elbow against your knee to facilitate the rotation. Hold for 30-60 seconds, switch legs, and repeat.

SAMPLE LESSON PLANS

Scope of the Lesson: Introduction to Stopping/Braking Technique

Sequence of the Lesson (45-minute class)

1. Introduce the importance of properly stopping/braking (5 minutes).
2. Warm-up exercises (5 minutes).
3. Demonstrate proper stopping/braking technique—teacher modeling (5 minutes).
4. Review key instructional cues for stopping/braking while demonstrating.

Figure 6.2   Hip and Back Stretch

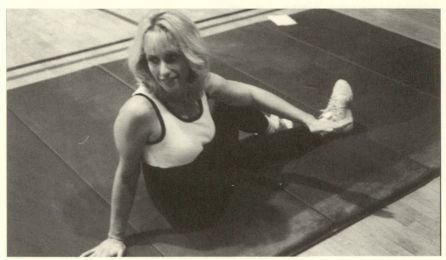

Photo by Matthew G. Butler

5. Review student checklist—"instructional cues" (5 minutes).

6. Allow for adequate student practice and individual instruction on stopping/braking (20 minutes).

7. Closure—general review of proper techniques/questions (5 minutes).

Major Skill Theme

Stopping/Braking

Instructional Cues

Preparing to Stop: The Ready Position

Skates several inches apart (almost touching) and parallel

- Face forward
- Knees slightly bent
- Look forward, not down

Stopping Technique:

- Roll braking skate forward, keeping the toe down
- When sliding braking foot forward, make sure it goes straight
- Line up in a straight line as if skating on a two-by-four
- Lift toe when braking foot is well in front of other foot (preferably at least 6 inches) before
- Bend knees to facilitate this action
- Keep back straight
- Braking foot should now be approximately 6 inches in front of the toe of other foot

- Keep weight on braking skate
- Keep center of gravity just behind the braking skate

Suggested Learning Activities

1. Teacher models proper stopping/braking technique and has students provide feed-back based on the instructional cues.

2. Students pair-up, observe, and assess their partner's stopping technique using the checklist as a guide (instructional cues). Students provide individual feedback to one another.

Teaching Styles

- Command Style for initial demonstration
- Individualized Instruction/Practice Centered (teacher observes each student as they execute stopping in front of the teacher)
- Reciprocal/Peer assessment utilized by students as they observe one another

TERMINOLOGY

ABEC: A scale, established by Annular Bearing Engineering Council, which measures the precision of a ball bearing, with ratings of ABEC-1, -3, -5, AND -7, with 7 being the most precise.

Aggressive Skating: Focus is on stunts, performed either on street courses or specially-built obstacles.

Anti-rockered: A wheel configuration in which the two middle wheels are smaller than front and back wheels on an in-line skate. This allows for grinds.

ANSI: American National Standards Institute. An organization which establishes standards for protective safety equipment.

ASTM: American Standards for Testing Materials. An organization which establishes standards for protective safety equipment.

Bearings: Mounted in pairs in the middle of each wheel. Bearings make in-line skate wheels turn easily.

Diameter: The width of a wheel as measured through its center. Measured in millimeters.

Durometer: The measure of a wheel's hardness. The scale ranges from zero to one hundred, hundred, with one hundred being hardest.

Frame: The portion of a skate which holds the wheels in place.

Freestyle: A variation of in-line skating that resembles figure skating. Also known as artistic skating.

Grind plate: A piece of metal (or plastic) attached to the bottom of the skate chassis between the middle wheels which allows for grinding.

Liner: The inner portion of the boot that cushions and supports the foot and ankle.

Profile: The thickness and shape of a wheel.

Recreational Skating: General skating.

Rockering: A wheel configuration in which the wheels are curved to improve maneuverability.

Rotate: To change the positions of in-line skate wheels to allow for even wear.

Snell: Foundation which tests and certifies helmets for safety reasons.

Spacer: A plastic or aluminum hub that separates bearing casings.

SELECTED READINGS

Dugard, M. (1996). *In-Line Skating Made Easy*. Guilford, CT: Globe Pequot Press.

Martin, J. (1994). *In-Line Skating*. Mankato, MN: Capstone Press.

Millar, C. (1996). *In-Line Skating Basics*. New York: Sterling Publications.

Nottingham, S. (1997). *Fitness In-Line Skating*. Champaign, IL: Human Kinetics.

Powell, M. (1997). *In-Line Skating*. Champaign, IL: Human Kinetics.

Rappelfeld, J. (1996). *The Complete In-Line Skater: Basic and Advanced Techniques, Exercises, and Equipment Tips for Fitness and Recreation*. New York: St. Martin's Press.

Savage, J. (1996). *In-Line Skating Basics*. Mankato, MN: Capstone Press.

7

Mountain Biking

THE NATURE OF MOUNTAIN BIKING

Mountain biking, also known as all-terrain or off-road biking, has grown tremendously over the last decade and is one of the best examples of a true lifetime sport. All-terrain bikes began appearing in the 1970's and participation has increased dramatically. Most people grow up learning how to ride a bike, and this activity offers the added adventure of exploring wooded trails and getting away from it all. Children learn to ride because it is fun; adults often continue to ride for basic transportation, fun, or the added benefit of developing their level of physical fitness. Many adults enjoy cycling and return to this activity because of the fun they had as a child. The beauty of mountain biking is that it can be done alone, with a friend or family, or as part of an organized cycling group.

Mountain bikes are able to take us on journeys that were never dreamed of and provide outdoor fun and enjoyment. In addition, cycling also provides us with another low impact activity.

INSTRUCTIONAL AREA

Basic instruction can occur in any number of places. In school settings, open parking lots are a good place to start for beginners as they learn to master the basics of shifting gears, turning, and stopping. This can naturally progress to local residential areas that are relatively free of traffic. Ideally, the next progression is to wooded trails. Many public school or university settings have trails that are located either on campus or in the local community. In addition, there are state, regional, and national biking trails located throughout the United States.

EQUIPMENT

Selecting a Bike

There are a number of models to choose from ranging from city bikes, which are a cross between a regular road bike and an all-terrain bike, true mountain bikes, and BMX-type racing bikes. These bikes all have a different set of specifications depending on their intended use. Frame geometry, tire type, and equipment are just some of the types of variations between each of these models.

Cycling enthusiasts will often refer to the "geometry" of a bike. This refers to the bikes dimensions, angles, lengths, and clearances of components such as the various tubes (steering, seat, vertical, and horizontal). Different types of bikes have different "geometry" depending on how they will be used.

Selecting the Proper Bike Size

Just as with selecting running and walking shoes, comfort is a key factor and a good indicator for the novice rider. There are some specific recommendations that will assist you in selecting the proper bike size.

The two most important factors in a perfect fit are seat height and distance between the saddle and the handlebars. Frame size, stem length, and stem height all affect these factors.

Frame Size: In general, the proper riding position consists of arms slightly bent with your back at a 45-degree angle to the ground. Many bikes allow your seat stem to be raised and lowered. Be sure that there is enough room (at least an inch) for your knees to rise up without hitting the handlebars. In choosing a bike, the frame size is the first consideration (sizes range from 16-23). The frame should be large enough to allow you to raise the seat to the appropriate height yet allow you to comfortably stand over the top tube with your feet flat on the ground. The frame size is too small if you need to raise the saddle above the minimum insertion line which may be found on the seat post. Another important consideration is the length of the frame. Select a frame that provides you with adequate room between your knees and the handlebars, otherwise you will be too cramped or your seated position will be too upright.

Top Tube Clearance: For safety purposes, mountain bikes require about 4-6 inches clearance between your seat and the top tube. This measurement is taken when you are standing with your feet flat on the ground.

Seat Height: To determine the proper seat height, sit on the bike with the cranks lined up with the seat tube. When you place your foot on the lower pedal, you should have about a one-inch bend in your knee.

Seat Position: Begin by sitting on the saddle (lean against a wall) with the cranks' parallel to the ground. Adjust the saddle position until your front knee is about 1-2 inches behind the pedal's axis.

Protective Equipment

1. Helmet—Snell approved or exceeds ANSI specifications
2. Biking shorts
3. Gloves
4. Mountain-biking shoes
5. Heavy cotton socks
6. Biking jersey
7. Eye protection
8. Windbreaker jacket and pants
9. Rearview mirror

Additional Equipment

Extra clothing is essential, especially if inclement weather is expected. As a minimum, you should bring a waterproof rain suit. If cold weather is expected, then bring along a synthetic jacket that continues to insulate even when it gets wet.

First Aid Kit

A first aid kit is essential, not only for yourself but to assist other riders who may fall. Small kits are available that can be stored on your bike or in a fanny pack.

Tools

For rides that remain close to home and are relatively short in duration, the standard compact mountain bike tool kit is adequate. These kits include such items as a chain tool, phillips and slot screwdrivers, allen wrenches, chain lube, crescent wrench, adjustable pliers, and a spoke wrench. You may want to include more equipment, especially if you plan a longer ride. Consider the following items, depending on the nature of your trip:

- Tire pump
- Patch kit
- Tire irons
- Spare tube
- Map and compass
- Sunscreen
- Lip balm with sunscreen
- Matches
- Swiss army knife
- Food and water
- Chain stay guard
- Toe clips
- Bike lock
- Headlight and taillight
- Fenders for inclement weather
- Reflective vest
- Panniers (storage bags strapped to your bike)

Maintenance

To ensure safety and to make your investment in your bike last, you should properly maintain your mountain bike. Your maintenance schedule will depend on how often you ride, but as a minimum, it is recommended that your bike be tuned up at least once a year. The following components of your bike need to be inspected and/or adjusted:

- Derailleurs
- Brakes
- Both wheels
- The hubs
- Bottom bracket and headset
- The tires for proper pressure
- All bolts
- General safety check

Do-it-yourself books can guide the novice through the maintenance process. However, it can be reassuring to have a professional bike shop care for your bike. In addition to the basic maintenance plan, it is recommended that a bike be totally overhauled every three years, especially if it is heavily used. This process basically entails dismantling the bike down to the frame, thoroughly cleaning it, and then rebuilding it. All spokes should be adjusted, and this is a good time to replace all cables. A waterproof bike grease should be applied to the bottom bracket, bearings, and headset to ensure smooth operation and optimal performance.

PROGRESSION

It is important for novice riders to limit their first rides on mountain bikes to the open parking lot. This will provide the teacher and new rider with an opportunity to learn the basics before heading out on an adventure which may eventually include rugged terrain and hills. Learning the basics of braking, shifting, and turning are essential for safety and developing self-confidence. In addition, short rides will help your body become physically accustomed to cycling, and this will help prevent muscle soreness.

After the basics have been mastered, the next natural progression is a short, off-road ride with a partner or group. Off-road terrain can be dangerous and should always be done with at least one other person. As you become more confident in your riding skills, you will naturally progress to more adventurous rides.

SKILLS AND TECHNIQUES

Learning to Stop

From a safety perspective, learning the proper way to stop your bike may be the most important skill and should be one of the first skills taught. In general, two fingers should be in contact with the brake levers. In more complicated situations on rough terrain one should always keep at least one finger on the brake lever. By maintaining a relatively loose grip on the brake lever you can dissipate some of the shock on the arms.

Approximately 60-70% of your braking capability comes from the front brake, however, using the front brake alone can be a recipe for disaster for novice riders. Sudden use of this brake, by itself, can cause the rider to be ejected over the handlebars. This type of accident can be avoided by (a) using both brakes, and (b) by keeping the center of gravity well back (do not lean forward while applying just the front brake).

Novice riders will have a natural tendency to be anxious which causes a rigid body position and a lot of body weight to be placed on the seat in a relatively stationary position. With guided practice, novice riders will learn to place more of their weight on their pedals and less on the saddle.

Shifting Gears

The primary reason for shifting gears is to effectively turn a multi-speed bike into the equivalent of a single-speed. Think of the front chain rings as fitting into two categories, low-range for hill climbing and high-range for flat terrain travel. Novice riders should be alerted to the importance of anticipating upcoming changes in terrain. They should shift the front derailleur before they reach the actual terrain ahead of them in anticipation of the change. Next, they will focus on the rear derailleur in which they will shift gears, as the terrain changes, under power. The center chainring can often be utilized for most of the varying terrain conditions that a rider will encounter. Using this method, the rider can simply use the range of gears in the rear derailleur. Anticipating changes in approaching terrain is essential for proper shifting and efficient riding.

Body Positioning and Balance

The most stable and desirable body position on a mountain bike consists of having your weight equally distributed on both feet, with level pedals, and the buttocks raised off of the saddle. Maintaining level pedals is critical to maintaining balance while going down hills as well as maximizing clearance over hazards. This position also allows the rider to easily adjust their center of gravity by leaning forward or backward as conditions dictate. This user-friendly position also makes riding more enjoyable because the knees can absorb the shock as opposed to the seat and spinal column.

Learning to Turn

Just prior to beginning a turn you should have your weight equally distributed on both feet, with level pedals, and the buttocks raised off of the saddle. Lean back slightly, depending on the terrain, and do most of your braking prior to entering the turn. You can then back off the brake as you continue the turn. A light touch on the brake should be maintained during the turn, and at the sharpest point in the turn braking should be minimal. As you complete the turn you will ease up on the brakes and may then move your weight forward slightly.

INSTRUCTIONAL CUES FOR RIDING

Uphill

- Do not spin the rear tire
- Keep constant pressure on the pedals
- Remain seated as long as possible
- Lean forward
- Keep elbows in
- Use the Bar ends

Downhill

- Pedals Level
- Place weight on pedals, not saddle
- Keep your weight back
- Tuck knees in
- Go slow
- Maintain slight braking to control speed
- Maintain a strong grip on the handlebars
- Absorb the shock with your elbows, knees, and hips

Clearing Small Obstacles

Learning the basic riding position, with weight on the pedals and buttocks off the saddle, provides the rider with a great position to learn how to clear small obstacles that they may encounter during a trail ride. This position will allow riders to move their center of gravity forward and backward on the bike in order to negotiate obstacles in rugged terrain.

The first step consists of learning to lighten and un-weight the front wheel. This is taught best without an actual obstacle. This lifting movement is accomplished by moving the bike out from under the rider by either moving the bike forward or by quickly moving your body weight backward. Once this has occurred, the next step is to move your body weight forward and straighten your legs once you are at the height of the obstacle. As the rear wheel contacts the imaginary obstacle, move your weight forward. This allows you to clear the obstacle without hitting it hard.

Trail Riding Etiquette:

The International Mountain Biking Association (IMBA) offers these guidelines for proper trail etiquette:

- Ride on Open Trails. Respect trail closures, private property, and requirements for permits and authorization. Federal and State wilderness areas are closed to cycling, and some park and forest trails are also off limits.
- Leave No Trace. Don't ride when the ground will be marred, such as muddy conditions after a rain. Never ride off the trail, skid your tires, or litter. Strive to pack out more than you pack in.
- Control your Bicycle. Excessive speed frightens hikers and may cause injuries which can result in trail closures.
- Always Yield. Make your approach known well in advance. A friendly greeting is considerate and appreciated. Show your respect when passing others by slowing to a walking speed or even stopping, especially in the presence of horses. Anticipate that other trail users may be around corners or in blind spots.
- Never Spook Animals. Give them extra room and time to adjust to you. Running livestock and disturbing wild animals is a serious offense. Leave ranch and farm gates as you find them, or as marked.
- Plan Ahead. Know your equipment, your ability, and the area in which you are riding, and prepare accordingly. Be self-sufficient at all times, keep your bike in good repair, and carry necessary supplies for changing weather conditions. Keep trails open by setting an example of responsible mountain biking.

FOCUS ON FITNESS

Trail riding has the potential to contribute to a number of the health-related components of fitness, specifically cardiovascular endurance, muscular strength and endurance, body composition, and flexibility. By focusing on long, slow rides, bikers can burn a significant number of calories which will help them improve their body composition by reducing body fat. Hill climbing will focus more on the development of muscular strength. As with running and walking, people who are interested in improving their cardiovascular fitness should monitor their heart rate to ensure they reach their training heart rate.

SAMPLE LESSON PLAN

Scope of the Lesson: Introduction to Riding, Learning to Turn

Sequence of the Lesson (45-minute class)

1. Introduce mountain biking as an excellent lifetime activity; explain how it increases cardiovascular fitness, muscular strength and endurance, and has social benefits (5 minutes).
2. Warm-up exercises (5 minutes).
3. Demonstrate proper turning technique—teacher modeling (5 minutes).

4. Review key instructional cues for turning while demonstrating.
5. Review student checklist—"instructional cues" (5 minutes).
6. Allow for adequate student practice and individual instruction on turning (20 minutes).
7. Closure—general review of proper turning techniques/questions (5 minutes).

Major skill theme

Proper Turning Technique

Instructional cues

- Prior to entering a turn
  - Have weight equally distributed on both feet
  - Level pedals
  - Buttocks raised off of the saddle
- Lean back slightly
- Do most of your braking prior to entering the turn
- Back off the brake as you continue the turn
- Maintain a light touch on the brakes (two fingers) during the turn
- Minimal braking at the sharpest point of the turn

Suggested learning activities

1. Teacher models proper turning technique and has students provide feedback based on the instructional cues.
2. Students' pair-up, observe, and assess their partner's turning form using the checklist as a guide (instructional cues). Students provide individual feedback to one another.

Teaching styles

- Command Style for initial demonstration
- Individualized Instruction/Practice Centered (teacher observes each student as they execute a turn in front of the teacher
- Reciprocal/Peer assessment utilized by students as they observe one another

TERMINOLOGY

Barends: An extension on the handlebars that is used for hill climbing.
Bottom Bracket: Mounts in the frame and holds the crank.
Brake Levers: Levers that are used to engage the brakes.
Cassette: Different sized cogs (7-8) on the rear hub that the chain utilizes to change gears.

Chain: The metal chain serves as a link and transfers the power of the pedal stroke to the rear wheel through the cassette and hub.

Chainrings: Chainrings are connected to the crank with most mountain bikes have 3 different chainring sizes for the chain.

Crank: The portion of the bike that contains the chainrings and pedals and is connected to the bottom bracket.

Derailleurs: This mechanism shifts the chain up and down the cogs or chainrings.

Frame: Series of hollow tubes which make up the main portion of a bike.

Headset: The mechanism that allows the front wheel to rotate.

Saddle: A bicycle seat.

Seatpost: A tube which attaches the frame and seat.

Spokes: Hold the hub and the rim together.

SELECTED READINGS

Nealey, W. (1992). *Mountain Bike: A Manual of Beginning to Advanced Technique.* Birmingham, AL: Menasha Ridge Press.

Toyoshima, T. (1995). *Mountain Bike Emergency Repair.* Seattle, WA: Mountaineers Books.

8

Volleyball

THE NATURE OF VOLLEYBALL

Volleyball provides people of all ages with a fun, non-contact, lifetime sport that can be played in a variety of ways. Young students can learn the fundamentals in middle school; high school and college students can play competitively; and adults can play either for fun or in competitive leagues. In addition, a cooperative version of the game can be played to lessen or eliminate the competitive aspect and foster cooperation and team-building.

INSTRUCTIONAL AREA

Indoor

Most instruction takes place on an indoor court in school settings. Because the equipment requirements are relatively low and easy to set up, volleyball is an ideal lifetime sport to be taught in school settings. Middle school students can begin the basics, and the learning process can continue through high school if a progressive sequence is planned.

Outdoor

The outdoor version, on grass or the beach, is popular among teens and adults. There are many variations of beach volleyball, which can be done with as little as two players on a side.

SKILLS AND TECHNIQUES

Forearm Pass

The forearm pass, also known as the underhand pass, is one of the first skills that new students should learn and that experienced students should review and continue to develop. The forearm pass is the method utilized when returning your opponents serve and is the critical link in transitioning from defense to offense. This basic skill is often called a "pass" when receiving the serve, and a "dig" when defending against your opponent's attack.

Footwork: Getting to the Ball

The first thing you must do is get to the ball. For balls that are hit relatively close to you it is important to move toward the ball without crossing your feet. Only when the ball is hit far from you should you use traditional cross-over running steps. In addition, anticipating where the ball is going to be hit by your opponent is critical. By focusing on this important aspect, you can attempt to get to the spot where you think the ball will land before it actually does.

The Ready Position

As with many sports, there are certain fundamental body positions that a student should be taught early on in the instructional process to set them up for success. For beginner students in volleyball, this basic position may be called the "ready" position. Once a student anticipates where the ball is going to land, and they get there, they must assume the proper body position prior to hitting the ball. This position consists of placing the feet shoulder width apart with one foot slightly in front of the other. The hands should be together with the thumbs facing forward and parallel and the elbows locked and the forearms rotated upward. The knees should be bent and arms extended out in front of the body so that they are parallel with the student's upper thigh. This parallel relationship will help you make contact with the ball down low, which is desirable. One of the most common errors, which leads to an inability to control the ball, occurs when beginning students attempt to pass the ball without first assuming the "ready" position.

Ready Position: Instructional Cues

- Arms straight and perpendicular to the upper body
- Bend at the waist
- Shoulders forward, hips back
- Knees bent

Contacting the Ball

Begin in the ready position and face the opponent who is hitting the ball over the net. It is very important, for control purposes, to always face the ball. As the ball approaches you, and just prior to contact, the student should extend their legs while simultaneously moving their arms in a slight forward and upward direction. The goal is to utilize the legs to power and control the ball as opposed to an arm action. Focus on the ball and watch it hit your forearms. After you contact the ball, it is important to follow through by continuing to move in the direction you want the ball to go by transferring your body weight to your front foot. This will greatly improve your ability to control the forearm pass. An important instructional cue is to always keep your arms lower than your shoulders.

Forearm Pass: Instructional Cues

- Assume the ready position
- Feet slightly more than shoulder-width apart
- One foot in front of the other
- Watch the ball contact forearms
- Extend the legs to propel the ball
- Follow through in the direction of the ball
- Keep arms below the shoulders at all times

Setting

The purpose of setting, also known as the overhand pass, is to place it in the proper position for a hitter to aggressively attack the ball to end the rally. The ball is normally "set" as the second contact after the forearm pass. There are a number of different paths the ball can take during the set including the "high outside" set, the "back" set, and the "quick" set, which is hit very low. The goal of the setter is to hit the ball vertically towards the outside of the court, about 8-10 feet in the air, so that it lands about 1-2 feet from the sideline. This places the ball in an ideal position for the attacker to hit the ball.

Preparing to Set: The Ready Position

Getting into proper position is critical in order to execute a proper set. The student should focus on bending the knees and place one foot in front of the other. The student should then place their hands in a diamond-shaped position and look between their hands at the approaching ball.

Figure 8.1   Volleyball Forearm Pass

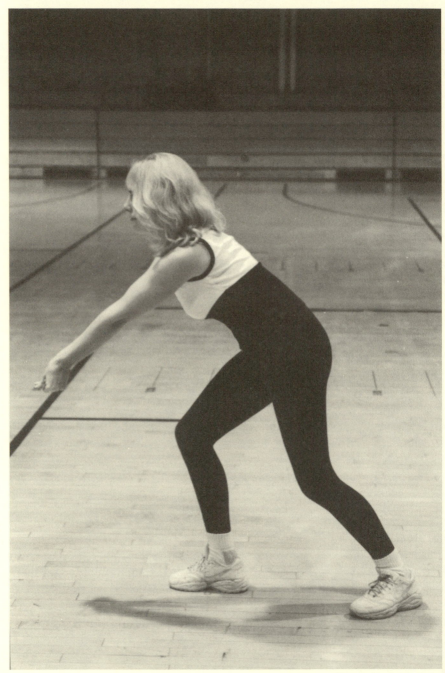

Photo by Matthew G. Butler

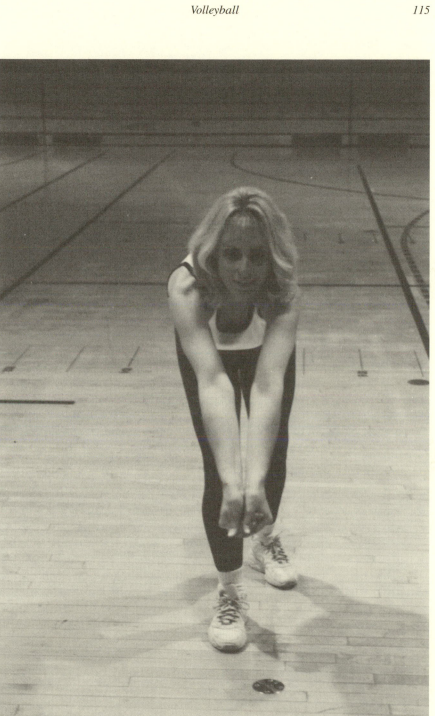

Photo by Matthew G. Butler

Contacting the Ball

A soft touch is used to contact the ball in setting. This is accomplished by placing the fingertips around the ball so that the hands mold to the shape of the ball. The fingertips wrapping around the ball helps maximize control. The actual hitting motion consists of extending the legs, wrists, and elbows in the direction of the intended target.

Instructional Cues: Setting

- Move quickly to the ready position
- Get under the ball
- Look through your hands at the ball
- Diamond-shaped hand position
- Fingertips contact the ball
- Extend arms, wrists, and elbows to contact the ball
- Follow through in the direction of the target

Serving

The "floater" serve is one of the most effective serves because the ball floats like a knuckleball weaving side to side in an unpredictable manner. New students can learn this serve by the numbers. Begin with preparing for a proper toss which is the foundation of a good serve. If you are right handed, hold the ball in front of your right shoulder with straight arms. Place your left hand on the bottom of the ball and your right hand on top. From this starting position, draw your right hand off the ball and bring your right elbow back and up. You will begin the actual serving motion when your hand is next to your head. As a self-check on the toss, you can toss the ball so it lands in front of your right foot. The height of the toss be about 6-8 inches higher than your extended right arm. As the toss nears its peak, begin your arm swing by extending your elbow and snapping at the ball. If the toss is not in the proper place, simply let it hit the ground and begin the sequence again. As with any many other sports, it is important to transfer weight from one foot to the other to gain power and momentum. You can accomplish this on the serve by stepping forward with your left foot as you contact the ball. One of the keys to getting the ball to "float" is to hit the ball with a stiff wrist, with the heel of your hand.

Serving: Instructional Cues

- Raise the ball in front of right shoulder
- Arms straight
- Right hand on top of ball, left hand on bottom

Figure 8.2   Volleyball Setting Position

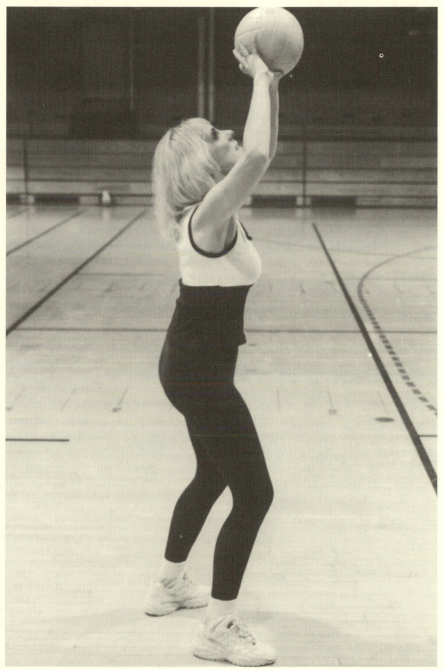

Photo by Matthew G. Butler

- Draw right hand back and elbow upward
- Toss ball 6 inches higher than your reach
- Step into the ball as you hit it
- Strike the ball with the heel of your hand, with a stiff wrist
- Move into a defensive position

Attacking (Spiking)

The hard spike is one of the most dramatic skills in volleyball and also the most challenging to master because it requires precise timing and coordination. If the initial hit—the forearm pass—and the second hit—the set—are hit correctly, the spike is the desired third and final hit by the offense.

Preparing to Spike

The starting position for the spike is near the attack line. The hitter should intently watch the setter to anticipate the direction of the set. The weight should be on the balls of the feet in a good athletic position. For right-handed hitters, the normal direction on the approach to the ball will be from left to right.

Spiking the Ball

Once the ball has been set, the hitter should begin their approach to the ball when the ball is at its highest point. Large steps should be taken in the approach with the last two steps closing together in order to transition to the jump. As the student jumps, both arms should raise up (forward) in preparation for the hit. The right arm should cock back and the left arm should point forward. The student should focus on hitting the ball directly in front of the right shoulder. The final action is to hit the ball with an open hand, on the palm area, and follow through the hit with a snapping action with of the wrist. Upon completion of the hit, the student must prepare for a safe landing by landing on both feet simultaneously, absorbing the landing by bending at the knees and hips.

Spiking: Instructional Cues

- Begin at the attack line
- Focus on the setter
- Weight on the balls of the feet
- Move forward when the ball reaches its highest point
- Take four large steps in the approach
- Close together on the last two steps
- Arms upward during the jump
- Right arm cocked, left pointing forward
- Hit the ball with your palm and snap the wrist
- Land safely on two feet with bent knees

Blocking

The key to effective blocking is anticipation. There are a number of clues that students should look for in order to determine the proper location to set up the block. The first clue is to watch the opponent's pass first pass. By observing them intently, students will be able to anticipate who the setter will be. Then, follow the ball and observe the setter's body position for the second hint as to where the ball will go next. Finally, by observing the hitters you will gain the final clue regarding the location and height of the set. Once you know where the ball is being directed, focus your attention on the hitter.

Getting in Proper Position: Footwork

The type of footwork that you utilize is determined by the distance that the student has to travel in order to get in blocking position. Normally, a student will only have to move about 5-7 feet to get in position. The step-close pattern should be utilized for this distance. This is accomplished by taking one large step in the direction of the ball, followed by a closing pattern with your opposite foot in preparation for the leap. If the set is to your left, then your left foot will step first and vice versa if the ball is to your right.

Blocking Technique

Jump as high as possible and focus on straightening your arms and pressing your shoulders against your ears. Once you have reached the highest point of your jump, spread your fingers as wide as possible and point your thumbs upward. At this point your should reach toward your opponent and angle your hands down in order to direct the ball towards the center. Once you have completed your blocking attempt, return to your normal position as quickly as possible.

Blocking: Instructional Cues

- Anticipate the proper blocking location
- Keep eyes open
- Jump as high as possible
- Fingers spread
- Think of wrapping your hands around the ball
- Arms against ears
- Direct the ball toward the center and downward

In most situations, three players should attempt to block the ball. The outside blocker's role is to correctly position the block. The outside blocker should be positioned inside the set, close to the sideline. This will take away the cross-court hit, yet cover the line. The role of the middle blocker is to cover all middle sets and to move towards the outside blocker to assist with an outside set.

COOPERATIVE GAMES

In the true spirit of lifetime sports, a cooperative version of volleyball can be played which eliminates the competitive aspect and focuses on cooperation, fitness, and recreational fun. This is a more social game which is very suitable for all ages and focuses on participation, not winning. Instead of having distinctly different teams, players rotate from one team to another during play. Instead of rotating out of play, players rotate to the other team.

FOCUS ON FITNESS

There are a number of strategies to promote the health-related components of physical fitness. With beginners in particular, normal six person volleyball may not promote fitness because the skill level may not be high enough for continuous activity to take place. One effective strategy is to reduce the number of players to four per team. This increases the activity of each student, allows for greater time on task, and will promote fitness due to greater activity.

SAMPLE LESSON PLANS

Scope of The Lesson: Introduction To Passing

Sequence of the Lesson (45-minute class)

1. Introduce the forearm pass as an essential, basic volleyball skill. (5 minutes).
2. Warm-up exercises (5 minutes).
3. Demonstrate the forearm pass—teacher modeling (5 minutes).
4. Review key instructional cues for the forearm pass while demonstrating.
5. Review student checklist—"instructional cues" (5 minutes).
6. Allow for adequate student practice and individual instruction on passing (20 minutes).
7. Closure—general review of proper passing techniques/questions (5 minutes).

Major Skill Theme

The Forearm Pass (Underhand pass)

Instructional Cues

Preparing for the forearm pass: The Ready Position

- Arms straight and perpendicular to the upper body
- Bend at the waist
- Shoulders forward, hips back
- Knees bent

Forearm Pass

- Feet slightly more than shoulder-width apart
- One foot in front of the other
- Watch the ball contact forearms
- Extend the legs to propel the ball
- Follow through in the direction of the ball
- Keep arms below the shoulders at all times

Suggested Learning Activities:

1. Teacher models proper passing technique and has students provide feedback based on the instructional cues.

2. Students pair-up, observe, and assess their partner's passing form using the checklist as a guide (instructional cues). Students provide individual feedback to one another.

Teaching Styles

- Command Style for initial demonstration
- Individualized Instruction/Practice Centered (teacher observes each student as they execute a pass in front of the teacher)
- Reciprocal/Peer assessment utilized by students as they observe one another

TERMINOLOGY

3-Meter line: The attack line.

Antenna: The flexible rod that is attached to the end of the net and designates the sideline boundary. It is considered part of the net and if a ball contacts the antenna it is out of bounds.

Back row: The three players near the baseline.

Baseline: The back boundary of the court (endline).

Block: Defensive players jumping in front of the opposing spiker to stop a spiked ball with the hands.

Bump: Forearm pass.

Dig: Successfully retrieving an opponent's ball close to the floor (pass).

Forearm pass: The basic skill that a player uses to hit the ball using the forearms.

Hitter: A player that is attacking.

Jump serve: An advanced serve in which the student jumps and attacks the ball similar to a spiking motion.

Kill: A ball that has been spiked and hits the floor or lands out of bounds after touching a defensive player.

Lift: A ball that remains in contact with a player for too long.

Post: The vertical standard that holds up the net.

Rally: A single series of play between two opposing teams that ranges from the serve until the ball is dead.

Serve: A fundamental skill (hitting the ball) that puts the ball in play.

Set: One of several basic skills, in which an overhead passing motion is utilized, to get the ball to a specific hitter who can then spike the hall.

Side-out: When the receiving team gains the serve due to an unforced error on the part of the serving team or when the receiving team hits the ball to the floor of the serving team.

Spike: A basic skill in which an attacker hits the ball aggressively into the opposing team's court.

Switch: A strategy in which two players change positions on the court after the serve.

SELECTED READINGS

Asher, K. (1997). *Coaching Volleyball*. Lincolnwood, IL: Masters Press.

Bertucci, R. (1993). *Volleyball Drill Book: Game Action Drills*. Lincolnwood, IL: Masters Press.

Howard, R. (1995). *An Understanding of the fundamental Techniques of Volleyball*. Needham Heights, MA: Allyn and Bacon.

Kilkenny, B. (1997). *Volleyball Rules*. New York: Sterling Publications.

Kiraly, K. (1999). *Beach Volleyball*. Champaign, IL: Human Kinetics.

Neville, W. (1989). *Coaching Volleyball Successfully: The USVBA Coaching Accreditation Program and American Coaching Effectiveness Program Leader Level Volleyball Book*. Champaign, IL: Human Kinetics.

Neville. W. (1994). *Serve it Up: Volleyball for Life*. Mountain View, CA: Mayfield Publishing Company.

Neville. W. (1990). *Coaching Volleyball Successfully*. Champaign, IL: Leisure Press.

Viera, B. (1996). *Volleyball: Steps to Success (Steps to Success Activity Series)*. Champaign, IL: Human Kinetics.

Wise, M. (1998). *Volleyball Drills for Champions*. Champaign, IL: Human Kinetics.

9

Tennis

———————————————————— *Karen Y. Peck*

THE NATURE OF TENNIS

Tennis is a game that people of all ages can enjoy. In addition to the opportunity to be active, many enjoy this game for the social interactions that it provides. For those who wish to participate at a competitive level, many tennis organizations utilize a skill rating system to ensure that players are well-matched and can enjoy good competition. At one time, tennis was a sport reserved for the wealthy, however, it has recently seen a huge increase in popularity. With that popularity has come an increase in the number of public courts and the opportunities for instruction and tournament participation at all levels.

INSTRUCTIONAL AREA

The rules of tennis state that a doubles court should be 78 feet long by 36 feet wide with a net that is 3 feet high in the middle and 3 1/2 feet high at the posts (figure 9.1). Tennis can be played indoors or outdoors and the game will vary slightly depending upon the venue. Outdoor players have to adapt to sunlight, darkness, wind, weather, and man-made distractions such as traffic or aircraft. Indoor players have to adapt to ceilings, lighting, and limited sideline space. Certain facilities also have huge "bubbles" which can be inflated during the winter months to transform an outdoor court into an indoor court.

There are a variety of surfaces on which tennis can be played. The three most common are asphalt, grass, and clay. Hard courts (asphalt or cement) are commonly seen at public facilities because they are easy and inexpensive to maintain. These courts may be fast or slow depending upon the materials used. Normally when these courts are constructed, sand is mixed into the surface paint,

Figure 9.1   Areas of the Court

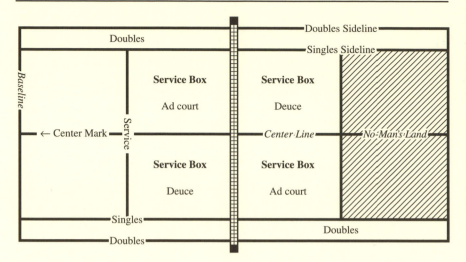

which grips the ball and slows it down as it bounces, preventing it from skipping across the surface. A court with more sand in the paint will be slower than one with less sand. Clay courts require a great deal of upkeep and are more expensive to maintain. A clay surface grips the ball causing the ball to bounce up and slow down. The accumulation of clay on the ball will cause it to become heavier as the match progresses. Grass courts are also very difficult and expensive to maintain. This surface is fast because the ball skips as it makes contact with the grass. The type of court surface determines the play of the ball and therefore the style and strategies employed by each player. A clay court match tends to have longer points and favors a player who prefers to stay toward the back of the court. A grass court match tends to have very short points and favors a player who prefers to rush the net.

Asphalt, clay, and grass are the most commonly used surfaces, but a teacher should not be limited to these three because tennis can also be played on such surfaces as carpet, turf, and rubber. A good teacher is aware of the rules of tennis but is not limited by them when teaching large groups of students. The game of tennis can be adapted to an infinite number of settings and surfaces in order to accommodate instruction.

EQUIPMENT

Tennis racquets come in a variety of sizes, materials, and prices. It is not necessary for a beginner to have an expensive racquet. Instead, it is important to start with a racquet that is light enough to control without elbow or wrist discomfort, and one that has a grip diameter that is appropriate for the player's hand size. A common method for determining grip size is to measure from the tip of the middle finger straight down to the first palm crease closest to the knuckles. This measurement, in inches, will correspond to the appropriate grip size.

Some racquets are sold pre-strung and others will need to be strung by a professional. A professional stringer can offer advice on the appropriate type of strings and the desired tension depending on the racquet, skill level, and playing style. In general, more string tension will offer less power but more control, and less string tension will offer more power but less control.

Tennis balls can be purchased inexpensively and should be replaced fairly often. Over time, they lose pressure and become "dead," which alters play.

Proper footwear is very important for a tennis player. The three most important considerations when selecting footwear are safety, comfort, and function. Footwear that is not designed for lateral movement, such as running shoes, can increase a player's risk of ankle and knee injuries. Select a shoe that is comfortable and designed for court use. In addition, some tennis facilities may have requirements pertaining to the sole of the shoe. Many shoes have dark, marking soles that leave a residue on the court surfaces. When the ball hits these marks it bounces or skips off the surface differently than it does on other areas of the court. Look for a shoe that has the label "non-marking sole." The shoe must allow for an adequate range of motion which promotes efficient stroke mechanics.

The most important consideration when choosing clothing is function. Consider the climate because lighter colored clothing reflects the sun's rays and is much cooler. Some facilities have a dress code requiring collars or prohibiting cut-off shorts. In general, follow the appropriate etiquette, and then choose clothing that is comfortable and functional.

Other accessories may help to make the game more enjoyable. Hats and sunglasses help protect the eyes from the sun and enhance vision. Sunscreen should always be used when playing outdoors, especially in the middle of the day, and sweatbands may help to keep your hands and face free from perspiration.

SKILLS AND TECHNIQUES

Spin and Grips

A key element to becoming a skilled tennis player is learning about spin and how it affects the trajectory of the ball. Skilled players are able to keep the ball inside the boundaries of the court by using spin to control the flight of the ball. A ball that is hit with topspin will pass a few feet above the net and drop down into the court. The key to producing spin is learning several racquet grips and using them with the appropriate stroke.

Hand placement on the racquet handle determines the angular orientation of the racquet face. A closed racquet face is one in which the strings are angled downward whereas an open racquet face is angled upward. The correct combination of racquet face orientation and stroke mechanics will keep the ball in play with spin. For example, when combining an open racquet face with a low to high stroke the ball will pass high over the net and land outside the court boundaries. However, when combining a closed racquet face with a low to high stroke, the ball will have topspin, which will cause it to pass a few feet over the net and drop down into the court.

There are three basic grips that all beginners should learn. These grips can best be learned by understanding the position, on the racquet handle, of the first knuckle of the index finger and the "V" of the hand formed by the thumb and index finger. There are eight flat surfaces, or bevels, on the grip of a racquet. These surfaces are described as the racquet is held with the strings perpendicular to the ground. (All grips are described for right-handed players. Left-handed players should shift their grip in the opposite direction.)

Continental Grip

When learning the continental grip, students should place the first knuckle on the first bevel to the right (at two-o'clock). The "V" of the hand should point toward the top bevel of the racquet. The continental grip is used for the slice serve, the overhead, and the volley.

Eastern Forehand Grip

When learning an eastern forehand grip, students should place the first knuckle on the bevel to the right that is parallel with the strings (at three o'clock). Point the "V" toward the first bevel to the right (at two o'clock). The eastern forehand grip is used for topspin forehand groundstrokes.

Eastern Backhand Grip

When learning an eastern backhand grip, students should place the first knuckle on the top bevel of the racquet that is perpendicular with the strings (at twelve o'clock). Point the "V" toward the first bevel to the left (at ten o'clock). The eastern backhand grip is used for topspin backhand groundstrokes.

Two-Handed Backhand Grip

When learning the two-handed backhand grip, students should start with a one-handed eastern backhand grip with the dominant hand. Place the non-dominant hand further up on the handle as if using an eastern forehand grip. Place the first knuckle of the dominant hand on the top bevel (at twelve o'clock) and the first knuckle of the non-dominant hand on the second bevel to the left (at nine o'clock). The "V's" of both hands point to the same bevel which is the first bevel to the left (at ten o'clock).

Figure 9.2   Continental Grip

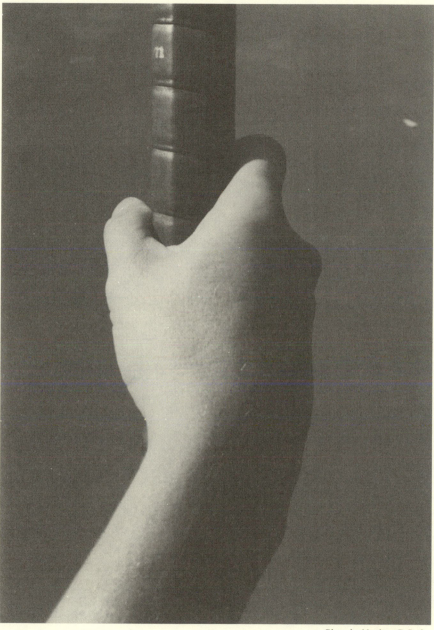

Photo by Matthew G. Butler

Figure 9.3   Eastern Forehand Grip

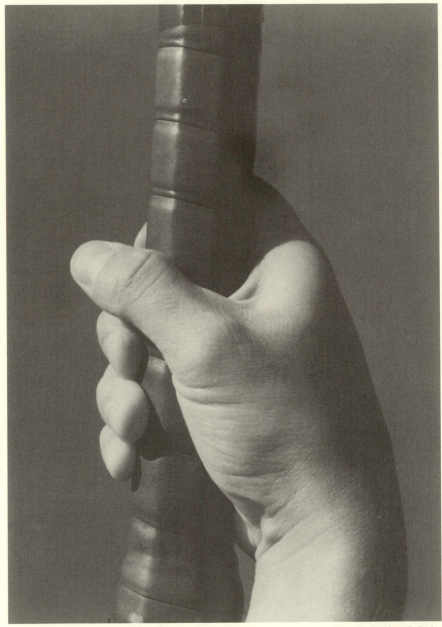

Photo by Matthew G. Butler

Figure 9.4   Eastern Backhand Grip

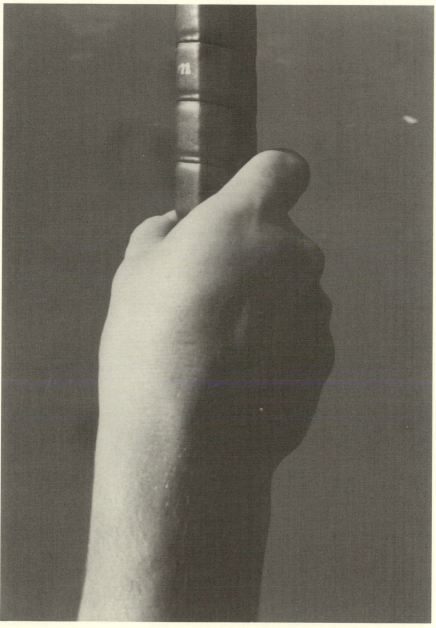

Photo by Matthew G. Butler

Figure 9.5   Two-handed Backhand Grip

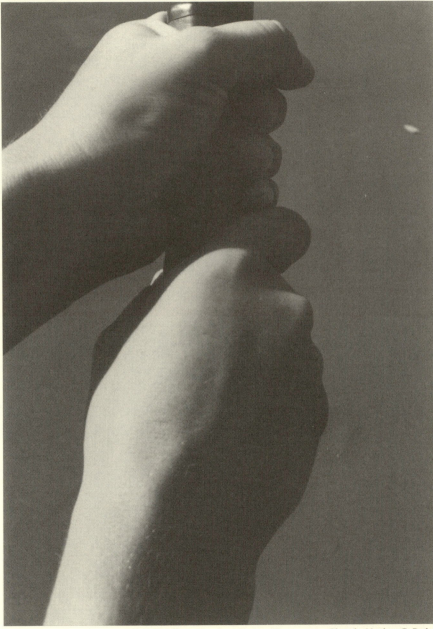

Photo by Matthew G. Butler

The Ready Position

Players should be in the "ready position" from the time that they finish a stroke until they begin to prepare for their next stroke. In the ready position, the player is on the balls of his or her feet, which are hip-width apart. The knees are bent and the player is leaning slightly forward at the waist. The racquet should be held in front of the player, perpendicular to the net, with the non-dominant hand supporting the throat of the racquet. A player in the ready position is able to efficiently move to any stroke on either the forehand or backhand side.

Instructional Cues: Ready Position

- Feet hip-width apart
- Weight on the balls of the feet
- Knees slightly bent
- Slight bend at the waist
- Racquet held out in front
- Support the racquet with the non-dominant hand

Forehand and Backhand Groundstrokes

Groundstokes are the foundation on which a tennis player's game is built. The player assumes the ready position at, or slightly behind, the baseline. The area of the court between the service line and a few feet inside the baseline is known as "no-man's land." It is in this area of the court that most balls bounce. A player standing in this area will have difficulty returning balls from this position because they bounce at his or her feet. By standing behind the baseline, the player receives the ball after the bounce when the ball is at a good height to hit a forehand or backhand groundstroke.

As soon as a decision is made as to which shot will be hit—forehand or backhand—the player quickly moves into position to receive the ball. When the player arrives at the position on the court where the ball will be played, he or she assumes a closed body position in order to receive the ball. A closed body position is one in which the body is facing the sideline and the opponent is unable to see the player's chest. This position allows the player to rotate the trunk as they swing the racquet, transferring more power to the shot. In contrast, an open body position is one in which the body stays facing the net forcing the player to extend the shoulder farther back to complete the stroke. The closed body position is recommended for beginners. As the player assumes the closed body position the racquet comes back early and the player remains on the balls of his or her feet. In this position, a player is able to make last minute adjustments necessitated by a gust of wind or a bad ball bounce. As contact is made with the ball, the weight of the body shifts to the front foot. Contact with the ball is made in front of the body which provides plenty of room between the body and the ball for a proper stroke.

Similar to batting in baseball, a player will get "jammed" if he or she receives a ball too close to the body. The player should keep his or her eye on the ball at all times, including the point in which the ball makes contact with the racquet.

A proper groundstroke has topspin that is created by a low to high stroke. The player brings the racquet back below the level of the shoulder, strokes through the ball, and follows through over the opposite shoulder. A closed racquet face moving from a low to high position creates topspin and sends the ball a few feet over the net and down into the court. The wrist remains stiff throughout the stroke. Topspin is imparted on the ball by a low to high stroke, not from a snap of the wrist. The wrist-snapping technique is not consistent and will create an increased risk of wrist and elbow injuries. In general, groundstrokes should land in the back half of the court because a ball that is hit deep keeps the opponent on the defensive and makes it more difficult for them to approach the net to volley.

Forehand Groundstroke

The forehand groundstroke is used when the ball is received on the dominant side of the body. For most players this is a more natural stroke to learn than the backhand. Beginners use the eastern forehand grip to execute a forehand groundstroke. This grip closes the racquet face when contact is made with the ball, allowing the player to stroke the ball from low to high and keeping it inside the baseline. At the end of the stroke, the follow-through brings the racquet up over the non-dominant shoulder.

Instructional Cues: Forehand Groundstroke

- Assume the "ready position"
- Eastern forehand grip
- Racquet back
- Non-dominant foot in front
- Closed body position
- Shift weight to front foot
- Stiff wrist
- Stroke low to high
- Contact the ball out in front
- Return to ready position

Backhand Groundstroke

The backhand groundstroke is used when the ball is received on the non-dominant side of the body. Beginning players should use the eastern backhand grip, which closes the racquet face, to facilitate topspin in the same manner as the forehand groundstroke.

The backhand can be one-handed or two-handed. A two-handed backhand is usually easier to learn than a one-handed backhand, but does not allow as much reach. This can limit a player's ability to return a wide ball.

Instructional Cues: Backhand Groundstroke

* Assume the "ready position"
* Eastern backhand grip (or two-handed grip)
* Racquet back
* Dominant foot in front
* Closed body position
* Shift weight to front foot
* Stiff wrist
* Stroke low to high
* Contact the ball out in front
* Return to ready position

Volley

A volley is a tennis shot in which the player hits the ball before it bounces. In general, the player will be at the net when using this shot. The continental grip is used for both the forehand and backhand volley, and because the player does not need to switch grips, there is more time to react quickly at the net.

The footwork of the volley is very important. As the player approaches the net from the baseline, he or she makes a split-step just as the opponent is making contact with the ball. A split-step is similar to the ready position with the feet equidistant from the net and hip-width apart. This position stops the player's forward momentum and allows him or her to make a quick move, either to the right or left, to receive a wide ball. When receiving a volley on the forehand side, the first step is a crossover step, with the non-dominant foot out in front of the body. This step allows for greater reach and forces the player to assume a more closed body position. Likewise, a crossover step in front with the dominant foot should precede the backhand volley. After each volley, the player returns to the ready position. In the ready position, the player holds the racquet in front of the body, perpendicular to the net, so that it is easy to go to the forehand or backhand side quickly. The player needs to be ready to volley, hit an overhead, or retreat backwards to return a ball that has been lobbed over his or her head.

As with the other strokes, the racquet comes back early, however, the volley has very little backswing. The racquet should not go past the plane of the body, the wrist is stiff, and the arm and racquet move as one unit from the shoulder. Players should meet the ball out in front of their bodies and "punch" the ball. The follow through only takes the racquet as far as the ready position. This stroke is always above the level of the net unless the ball was received lower than the level of the net. It is important that the racquet head always remain above the wrist. In the event that the ball is received very low, the player bends at the knees and maintains a very low body position to keep the racquet head above the wrist.

The player's momentum should always move toward the net unless he or she is retreating to chase down a lob. Hit volleys deep so that your opponent remains in a defensive position and eventually is unable to return a quick, hard-hit volley. The effectiveness of a volley comes from the quick return and deep placement of the ball, not from a big swing.

Instructional Cues: Volley

- Assume the "ready position"
- Continental grip
- Short back swing
- One step toward the ball
- Meet the ball out in front
- Stiff wrist
- Punch the ball
- Follow through to the ready position

Serve

The serve is the only stroke in tennis in which a player has complete control of the stroke from start to finish. There are three basic types of serves to include: the flat serve, the slice serve, and the topspin serve. I recommend that the slice serve be taught to beginners because it is easy to learn and it is a high percentage serve.

Begin by reviewing the continental grip, which is used for the slice serve. Next, have the player assume an upright body position with the non-dominant foot at a 45-degree angle to the target. At no time during the serve can the player's foot touch the baseline or any part of the court inside the baseline.

The most important part of the serve, and the part in which most mistakes are made, is the toss. A good toss has no spin. It may be easier to think of the toss as a "lift." The ball is lifted up using the palm of the hand and not the fingers. It should reach a height equaling at least the height of the racquet with the arm fully extended. If the toss is correctly placed, the ball will land on the ground approximately twelve inches in front of the dominant foot. Consistency of toss placement is key. After the toss, the non-dominant hand remains extended with the hand pointed toward the ball. Maintaining this position will ensure that the non-dominant shoulder does not drop and that the shoulders do not prematurely rotate. This also helps to add consistency to the serve. The backswing brings the racquet into a "back scratch" position where the racquet is over the shoulder but angled so that it is almost touching the back. From this position, the player simply extends the arm upward so that the racquet makes contact with the ball approximately twelve inches in front of the body, over the dominant shoulder, extended upward so that contact is made at the highest possible point. The follow through of the racquet is in front of the body and the momentum of the stroke should carry the entire body into the court.

Instructional Cues: Serve

- Continental grip
- Body angled 45 degrees to the target
- Ball toss ("lift") at least as high as the reach of the racquet
- Non-dominant hand points toward the ball
- Back scratch
- Contact the ball high
- Hit down into the court
- Return to ready position

Figure 9.6   Serve: Ready Position

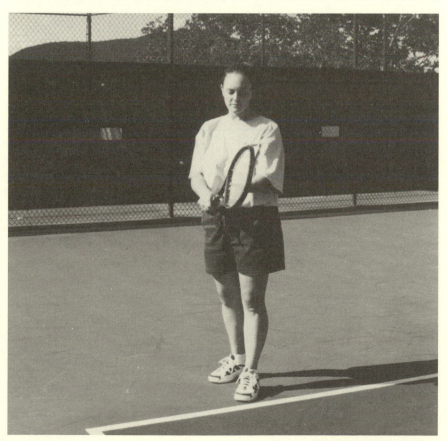

Photo by Matthew G. Butler

Figure 9.7   Serve: Ball Toss

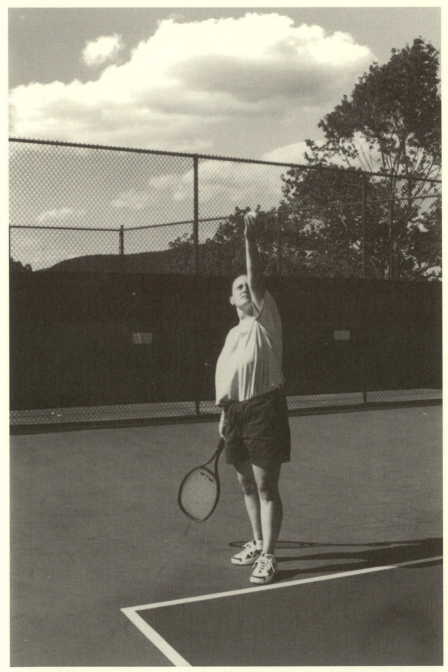

Photo by Matthew G. Butler

Figure 9.8   Serve: Back Scratch Position

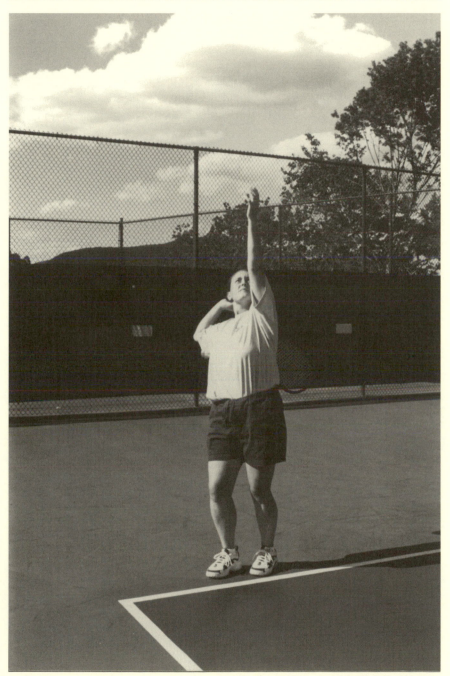

Photo by Matthew G. Butler

Figure 9.9   Serve: Ball Contact

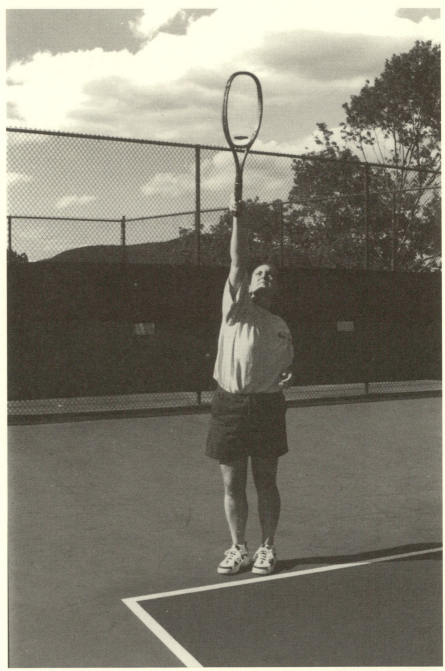

Photo by Matthew G. Butler

Overhead

The overhead shot is used when the opponent hits a lob that passes high over the net and slowly comes back down into the court. An overhead shot is a good opportunity to win a point because the ball can be hit very hard down into the court, which is difficult for the opponent to return.

The overhead shot uses the same motion as the serve. Using a continental grip, get into a good court position to hit the ball, keeping in mind that the ball is contacted in the same place as it would be for a serve. When in position, the body should be at a 45-degree angle to the target, the non-dominant hand is pointed toward the ball, and the racquet is in the "back scratch" position. Make contact with the ball at the highest point possible with the arm fully extended.

Instructional Cues: Overhead

- Continental grip
- Body is at a 45 degree angle to the target
- Assume the "back scratch" position
- Point non-dominant hand toward ball
- Contact the ball as high as possible
- Snap the wrist
- Hit the ball down into the court
- Return to the ready position

Lob

The lob is a shot that is hit very high over the net and slowly drops down into the court. A lob can be used to pass an opponent who is at the net or to change the pace of the point. The technique of the lob is very similar to a groundstroke. The difference is in the racquet face angle and racquet head speed. The ready position, grip, and preparation are the same as the forehand or backhand groundstroke. When making contact with the ball, open the racquet face slightly. Also, slow down the speed of the racquet head slightly. By making these two changes, the ball passes much higher over the net and drops deep into the court. Strive to hit the ball deep into the court to avoid giving your opponent an opportunity to receive an overhead close to the net.

Instructional Cues: Lob

- Assume the "ready position"
- Use the eastern forehand or backhand grip
- Racquet back—open the racquet face slightly
- Closed body position
- Swing low to high
- Slower racquet head speed than groundstrokes
- Return to the ready position

Scoring

The scoring system in tennis consists of points, games, sets, and matches. A point consists of one rally between players that ends when one player fails to return a ball before the second bounce or within the boundaries of the court. A player must win four points, by a margin of at least two, in order to win a game. The points are called love—zero points, 15—one point, 30—two points, 40—three points, and game—four points by a margin of at least two. For example, if the server won the first three points and lost the fourth point the score would be 40–15. When the score is tied at four points each, or 40–40, the score is called deuce. The next player to win a point is said to have the advantage or "ad." If the same player wins the next point he or she wins the game. However, if that same player loses the next point the score returns to deuce and the game continues.

A player must win six games, by a margin of at least two, to win a set. Many tournament formats call for a tiebreaker to be played when the score is at six games each. In a tie-breaker, players take turns serving two points at a time and continue until one player has won seven points, by a margin of at least two points. Instead of the scoring system described earlier (love, 15, 30, etc.) numerical scoring is used for tiebreakers. The winner of the tiebreaker is the winner of the set and the score of that set is called 7–6. In general, men must win three out of five sets and women must win two out of three sets in order to win the match.

This scoring system is commonly used in professional tournaments. There are, however, a number of different formats that are used in tournament play. For example, some matches consist of a ten game set in which only one set is played and the winner must win ten games by a margin of two. Some tournaments do not use tiebreakers in the final set. Instead players continue indefinitely until one player has won by a margin of at least two games. Other tournaments use no-ad scoring. In this type of play, the first player to win four points is the winner of the game whether it is by a margin of four points or one point (see selected readings for further explanations of scoring and rules).

Strategy

The strategy employed by each player should be determined by his or her strengths and weaknesses, the opponent's strengths and weaknesses, the playing surface, and the conditions. There are two predominant styles of play, and within those two styles exist great differences among players. A "baseliner" tends to stay back at the baseline and hit groundstrokes. A "serve and volleyer" takes every opportunity to come up to the net and volley, oftentimes doing so immediately after their own serve. The surface of the court often gives advantage to a certain style of play. A slower court, such as clay, favors a baseliner, whereas a faster court, such as grass, favors the serve and volleyer.

Acquiring tennis skills requires a good teacher and a lot of practice. A style of play, on the other hand, is hard to teach and only develops over time and with experience. However, there are some basic concepts that apply to any tennis game that can be taught to beginners to help them develop their own strategies and styles of play.

In general, when less skilled players compete against each other, the player who makes the fewest errors and keeps the ball in play will win. Many beginners aim for the lines and try to hit the ball too hard without control and end up losing points. Players should analyze and take advantage of their opponent's weaknesses. For example, many beginners have a weaker backhand than forehand. To take advantage of this weakness, hit more balls to the backhand. In addition, get the first serve in play whenever possible. Many players hit the first serve hard, without control, and do not place many inside the service box. This serve is usually followed by a cautious, weak second serve that gives an advantage to the opponent. Take a little pace off the first serve and get more in play. Likewise, take advantage of an opponent who misses a lot of first serves by being aggressive and stepping into the court a few steps before the second serve.

If a player is a good volleyer, they should take every opportunity to approach the net and win the point. A good time to approach is when the opponent has been forced to play deep in the court or in the corners. If the opponent hits a short ball in the middle of the court, hit the ball and continue moving up to the net to volley the next ball. If the opponent is at the net, hit a passing shot down the sideline to force a stretch, or lob the ball deep into the court to force a retreat back to the baseline.

Etiquette

Etiquette is a set of unwritten rules which facilitates the flow of play, enables unfamiliar players to play together comfortably, and ensures fair play. It is every player's responsibility to understand these unwritten rules of etiquette that govern tennis play.

Tennis is a unique game in that only the highest level of competition utilizes referees. Many collegiate and community sponsored events do not have referees or only have one referee to supervise several matches. For this reason, it is important for players to be aware of the rules and etiquette to maximize the enjoyment for all players. The following is an overview of tennis etiquette and may not be all-inclusive. For a complete guide to etiquette and rules, refer to the selected readings section.

Before each point, the server should call out the score—calling the server's score first—in order to avoid disagreements later in the match. The server should always begin the point with possession of two balls in order to ensure a good flow of the game. Never cross another court in the middle of a point. If a ball accidentally crosses your court, a "let" should be called and the point replayed. Each player should make the calls on their own side of the net immediately after the point. If there is a question about the call, the point should go to the opponent. Spectators should remain quiet during all points and keep movements to a minimum.

The nature of tennis officiating is a perfect opportunity to teach students the value of fair play. This game is enjoyable only if you follow the rules and proper etiquette. Players who consistently disregard these rules have trouble finding, and keeping, opponents and doubles partners.

FOCUS ON FITNESS

Tennis can be an enjoyable way to maintain a level of physical fitness throughout life. The level of fitness that is demanded is dependent upon the setting in which the game is played. A singles match played on a clay court is likely to require more endurance than a doubles match played on a hard court. Many tennis enthusiasts participate in tennis drill sessions or footwork drills at local clubs or parks, which can be much more physically demanding than simply rallying back and forth with a partner.

Attaining a basic level of fitness is advisable for anyone attempting to learn to play tennis. Players should develop their cardiorespiratory endurance and flexibility as well as their basic movement skills to include agility and hand-eye coordination. Players who want to develop their game further will need to focus on areas of fitness specific to tennis. Tennis is a game of inches, and a player who is highly skilled, but not in good physical condition, will not fare as well on the court. Tennis is an anaerobic sport comprised of very short, intense points followed by periods of recovery. A workout session should closely resemble these intervals. However, aerobic conditioning should not be neglected as many tennis matches can last 4 hours or more. A muscular strength and flexibility program should be incorporated into the fitness regimen to assist with injury prevention. Sport-specific drills should be interspersed within this fitness plan to improve agility, quickness, and reaction time. In addition, every practice session should begin with a sport-specific warm-up and end with a good cool-down.

Good footwork is an important asset for any tennis player. A good forehand will go to waste if a player cannot get their body in the correct position to use it. Good footwork should be incorporated into every tennis drill. For example, when practicing the volley, players should run back to the service line in between each shot. This will force the player to make a split-step before each volley and will also make the drill more physically demanding. When practicing overheads, the players should run up to the net in between each shot because many overheads are hit while retreating from the net. Adding components of footwork into each drill will more closely simulate game play and will give students a more challenging work out.

TEACHING LARGE GROUPS

Teaching tennis to a large group of students may seem daunting at first. Due to the size of the court and the number of players able to play at once, there can be a lot of down time for most of the class. However, a good educator can make modifications to the game in order to adapt it to any facility with any number of students. The key is to be creative with the resources that are available and to get the whole class involved and engaged in playing.

Safety Considerations

Before teaching tennis or any other activity, it is important to take a look at safety issues for the specific facilities, equipment, and lesson plans. First, always make sure the teaching environment and the equipment are safe. For example, when racquet handles are in poor condition, it is possible for players to lose their grip during a stroke and the racquet can hit another player. Shoes should be selected which provide support for the lateral movements required by tennis. Teaching proper techniques will reduce the occurrence of overuse injuries such as wrist strains and tennis elbow. When organizing the lesson plan, make sure that all drills have a built-in system for ball retrieval. Students should be responsible for ensuring that no stray balls are on the court that can cause injury to other players. And finally, beginning students should have a basic level of fitness before learning a new sport. Tennis demands endurance, hand-eye coordination, and agility. Possessing these skills prior to stepping on the court will decrease the risk of injury. As with all other physical activities, a good warm-up, cool-down, and stretching session is always important in order to reduce the risk of injury.

SAMPLE LESSON PLAN

This lesson is designed for 40 high school students and two tennis courts, or a space that is equivalent in size. The equipment that is needed includes 20 racquets, 25 tennis balls, 20 pencils, and 40 instructional cue worksheets. Many substitutions can be made if equipment is not available. For example, racquetballs can be used instead of tennis balls.

Scope of the Lesson: Introduction to the Volley

Sequence of the Lesson (45-minute class)

1. Warm-up and stretching (5 minutes).
2. Tennis warm-up drill—racquet- and ball-handling (10 minutes).

   - 20 students at a time are inside a square or a set of boundaries clearly marked on the floor. Each student has a racquet and a ball (the other 20 students stand outside the boundaries and act as referees and retrieve lost balls outside the boundary).
   - Each student inside the square bounces the ball up in the air with the racquet while the other students try to take the ball or swat it away. Students may only

touch the ball and may not touch other racquets or other students. As soon as a
student loses their ball they exit the square.
- The game continues until only one student remains.
- The two groups of students switch places.
- Variation two: Students can bounce the ball against the ground with the racquet
instead of up in the air.

3. Discuss the volley and when it is used in the game of tennis (2-3 minutes).
4. Demonstrate the volley using the instructional cues—teacher modeling (5 minutes).
5. Form groups of four. Two students stand approximately 10 feet apart and volley
back and forth keeping the ball above the level of an imaginary net. The goal is to
get as many touches in a row as possible in a cooperative manner, not to "beat" the
opponent. The other two students should provide feedback using the student checklist with instructional cues. After five minutes, the volleyer's switch places with the
"teachers" (10 minutes).
6. In the same groups of four, see which pair can get the most touches before the ball
touches the ground (5 minutes).
7. Provide effective closure: review the lesson and the instructional cues (2-3 minutes).
8. Cool down and stretching (5 minutes).

Major Skill Theme

The Volley

Instructional Cues

Preparing for the volley: The Ready Position

- Feet hip width apart
- Weight on the balls of the feet
- Knees slightly bent
- Slightly bent at the waist
- Continental grip
- Racquet held out in front
- Support the racquet with the non-dominant hand

Volley

- Short backswing
- One step toward the ball
- Meet the ball out in front
- Stiff wrist
- Punch the ball
- Follow through to the ready position

Teaching Styles

- Direct instruction occurs as the teacher introduces and teaches the volley.
- Teacher provides individual and group-directed feedback during the volley practice session.
- Students use an instructional cues worksheet and provide peer/reciprocal teaching (be sure that students have been instructed on how to provide effective feedback to their peers).

Safety Considerations

- Prior to class, make sure that all equipment and facilities are in good working order and the instructional area is safe.
- Instruct students in the proper warm-up and cool-down techniques.
- During the tennis warm up drill, instruct students to immediately retrieve the balls so that no other student steps on them.
- During the volley practice session, ensure that each team of four is adequately spaced so that no one is in danger of being hit by the swing of a racquet.

Other Suggestions for Lesson Plans

Tennis is a perfect game to teach in conjunction with math skills. Younger students can learn by completing a task to measure the dimensions of a tennis court. Higher level students can be challenged to examine angles and margin of error. For example, how does a higher contact point on a serve change the angle of the ball into the court, and therefore the margin of error? How does spin alter these margins? (see selected reading)

TERMINOLOGY

Ad court: As a player is facing the net, the service box to the left on the same side of the net, or the right on the opposite side of the net.

Alley: Area of the court between the singles sideline and the doubles sideline.

Approach Shot: A ball that is played immediately before a player comes to the net, with the intent of forcing a weak return from the opponent.

Backcourt: Area of the court between the service line and the baseline.

Backhand: Stroke used when the ball is received on the non-dominant side of the body.

Baseline: Endline, or the boundary of the court farthest from the net.

Canadian doubles: Match play involving a team of two players against one other player. The team of two players must place their shots within the singles sideline. The lone player may hit within the doubles sidelines.

Closed racquet face: The contact surface of the strings is angled downward.

Closed stance: Body position in which the player's chest is facing the sideline rather than the net.

Continental grip: Hand position on the racquet used for the slice serve, volley, and overhead.

Deuce court: As a player is facing the net, the service box to the right on the same side of the net, or the left on the opposite side of the net.

Doubles: Match play in which four players participate on one court as teams of two.

Doubles sideline: Line perpendicular to the net outside the singles sideline, which forms the outside boundary for doubles match play.

Drop volley: A ball that is played out of the air and lands short in the opponents court, making it difficult for an opponent standing at the baseline to return.

Drop shot: A groundstroke that lands just over the net and is difficult for an opponent standing at the baseline to return.

Eastern backhand grip: Hand position on the racquet handle used for the backhand groundstroke.

Eastern forehand grip: Hand position on the racquet handle used for the forehand groundstroke.

Flat serve: Serve delivered with little or no spin.

Foot-fault: If on the serve, the foot touches the line or any part of the court inside the line before the racquet makes contact with the ball.

Forehand: Shot played when the ball is received on the dominant side of the body.

Grip: Hand position on the racquet that determines the racquet face angle.

Groundstroke: Shot played after the bounce from the backcourt.

Half-volley: A shot in which the ball is contacted immediately after the bounce.

Let: An interruption in play demanding that the point or the serve be replayed.

Lob: A ball that is hit with a great deal of arc with the intention of changing the pace of the point or of passing over the opponents head as they stand at the net.

Mixed Doubles: Each doubles pair consists of one male and one female.

No-man's land: Area of the court between the service line and a few feet inside the baseline.

Open racquet face: The contact surface of the strings is angled upward.

Open stance: Body position in which the player's chest is facing the net rather than the sideline.

Overhead: A shot in which contact with the ball is made high in the air and the ball is hit hard down into the opponent's court.

Passing shot: A shot that is hit past an opponent who is moving toward or standing at the net.

Ready position: Position assumed as the player is waiting to receive the ball.

Serve: A shot that initiates every point and must land in the opponent's service box.

Serve-and-volley: A style of play in which a player's intent is to get in a position at the net in order to volley.

Service line: Line parallel with the net in between the net and the baseline, which forms the back boundary for the service box.

Singles sideline: Line perpendicular to the net inside the doubles sideline that forms the outside boundary for singles match play.

Slice: See Underspin.

Split-step: A ready position that prepares a player to hit a volley after approaching the net from the baseline.

Throat of the racquet: Area of the racquet between the grip and the racquet head.

Tie-break: A series of points played at the end of a tied set, which will decide the winner of that set.

Topspin: The top surface of the ball rotates against the air resistance creating increased friction, causing the ball to drop faster than if it had no spin.

Underspin: The bottom surface of the ball rotates against the air resistance creating increased friction, causing the ball to be lifted and stay up in the air longer than if it had no spin.

Volley: A ball that is played in the air before hitting the ground.

SELECTED READINGS

Douglas, P. (1992). *The Handbook of Tennis*. New York: Alfred A. Knopf.

Gallwey, T. (1997). *The Inner Game of Tennis*. New York: Random House.

Hoskins, T. (1997). *1001 Incredible Tennis Games, Drills and Tips: A Super Abundance of Information for Every Teaching Professional and Tennis Enthusiast*. Somerset, NJ: Hoskins Publishing.
http://www.bookmaster.com/marktplc/00249.htm

Metzer, M. Sebolt, D. (1994). *Interactive Learning Approach: Student Personal Workbook for Tennis*. Dubuque, IA: Kendall/Hunt Publishing Company.

Vasquez, R. (1997). *Kid's Book of Tennis: Over 150 Games to Teach Children the Sport of a Lifetime*. Secaucus, NJ: Carol Publishing Group.
The Rules of Tennis
Official Code of the International Tennis Federation
http://www.littletennis.com
http://wings.ucdavis.edu/Tennis/index.html

SPORT SPECIFIC ORGANIZATIONS

United States Professional Tennis Association
USPTA World Headquarters
3535 Briarpark Drive Houston, TX 77042
(800) USPTA-4U (877-8248) or (713) 978-7782
FAX (713) 978-7780
http://www.uspta.org

United States Tennis Association, Inc.
70 West Red Oak Lane
White Plains, NY 10604-3602
(800) 990-8782
http://www.usta.com

10

Swimming

By Raymond J. Bosse

THE NATURE OF SWIMMING

Swimming is an ideal lifetime sport because it contributes to several of the health-related components of fitness, namely, muscular endurance, flexibility, and cardio-vascular fitness. It is a great choice because people may participate either alone or in groups, and the fact that it is done in the water eliminates the impact injuries to joints that other activities can cause. In addition, many communities have facilities that will enable your students to enjoy swimming either indoors during the winter or outdoors during the warmer months. Swimming can be done at your own pace and helps to relieve stress while exercising almost every muscle in the body. These unique factors allow individuals to continue to enjoy the activity well into their 80's or beyond! The proliferation of Master's Swim Clubs around the world is a testament to the growing popularity of the sport, and there are over 37,000 registered master's swimmers in the United States alone! In addition to providing the adult swimmer with a place to share their desire for health and fitness, masters clubs also serve as an important social center. Going to the pool is no longer just an activity for the kids!

Swimming also serves as a gateway to several similar aquatic sports such as scuba diving, water polo, and triathlons. These sports are more easily learned if a student has a basic swimming background.

Many students learn basic "survival swimming" skills at a young age which enable them to enter the water without a fear of drowning. Most students, however, have not been taught the specific skills which will allow them to participate in swimming as a mode of exercise. These specific skills can be taught to basic level swimmers.

EQUIPMENT

Swim Suits

A functional swimming suit is an essential piece of equipment in order to enjoy swimming. There has been a proliferation of materials and designs in recent years which may confuse consumers. A suit should be comfortable, yet light in weight in order to avoid excessive drag. The most common suit is also one of the best—the nylon swim suit. This suit is recommended for beginners because of its durability. This durability can be increased even more if the suit is rinsed in clean water after each use to remove the chlorine. Racing suits are made from a variety of lycra materials that are more expensive, specifically designed for advanced racers, and not as durable.

In general, a suit should be form fitting. For women, I recommend a one-piece suit that allows for complete rotation of the shoulders and adequate support of the bust. Most sporting goods stores have a selection that will meet the needs of the average swimmer.

There are several types of garments that should be avoided. Men should avoid large baggy suits and cut-off jeans because they cause the hips to sink, and make efficient swimming difficult. Two-piece suits for women should be avoided unless they are specifically designed for fitness swimming.

Goggles

I recommend that new swimmers wear goggles because they prevent the pool chemicals from irritating students' eyes. In addition, goggles reduce the natural apprehension that many young swimmers have about placing their face in the water. Reducing this apprehension can enhance the student's ability to learn.

Goggles range in price from $3.00 to $15.00, but before buying a pair I recommend you try a friend's pair. Everyone's face is different, and goggles that fit one person well may not fit another. The two key factors in selecting goggles are comfort and the ability of the goggles to keep your eyes dry. If you swim both indoors and outdoors, consider buying two pairs—one for indoor use and a dark pair to reduce the glare of the sun. Goggles should have individual eyepieces and be padded with foam or rubber for comfort to insure a proper seal around the eyes. Many new swimmers find the foam-padding version to be the most comfortable. Most sporting goods stores will carry a basic supply of goggles, but there are also stores that deal strictly with swimming apparel. These stores can be located in swimming and triathlon magazines or on the Internet.

Swim Caps

Swim caps are a matter of personal preference and are often considered a necessity by people with long hair. There are three basic types of caps; latex, lycra, and silicon. The latex cap is the most popular, fits the needs of most recreational swimmers, and costs between $3.00 and $5.00. Lycra caps do not keep the hair as dry as the silicon cap, which is more expensive. The life of all caps can be increased by drying them thoroughly and sprinkling them with baby powder after each use.

Training Aids

There are a number of training aids that are available for swimming with the most common being kickboards, pullbouys, fins, and paddles. The problem with some of these devices is that they can actually inhibit the development of proper body balance. A new item called "fist gloves" may be useful in teaching the important concept of proper body position. These latex gloves are molded into a fist which greatly reduces the hand's ability to provide propulsion.

SWIMMING SAFETY

Swimming is an activity which has obvious risks, and in order to manage this risk I recommend that teachers follow these safety guidelines:

- Always swim in a designated swimming area that has certified lifeguards.
- Insure proper hydration. Hydrate before, during, and after swimming. Even though your students are in the water, they still need to replace fluids.
- Use sunscreen when swimming outside. The water reflects the sun's rays, and a 30 minute swim outdoors can result in a severe burn.
- Be alert for ear infections. Regularly flushing the ears with isopropyl alcohol after swimming and showering can help prevent infection. If you develop pain, stop swimming and consult a physician.
- If you feel any type of pain, stop swimming immediately and seek medical care.

Warm-up

The warm-up and cool-down phases described in Chapter 4 are also applicable for swimming, and the stretches described for running are also appropriate for swimming.

SWIMMING SKILLS AND TECHNIQUES

The freestyle stroke is the most common of the 4 swimming strokes and the primary choice of people who swim for fitness. There are three principles that can help the novice swimmer become more efficient in the water. These principles are include "proper balance" in the water, "swimming tall," and swimming by "skating" on your side. These three principles all rely on proper body position.

Body Position

The most important aspect of swimming is to learn the basic body position. This consists of achieving a level position on the surface of the water from your head to your toes. This is learned by gently kicking short distances with the hands at the side and the eyes looking at the bottom of the pool. This is called "hiding your head" and is essential in learning proper body position. The head should be in line with the body and the eyes should be focused on the bottom of the pool, not forward.

As you can see in Figure 10.1, if the head is raised, the hips and legs are forced down in the water resulting in an unbalanced body position. By keeping the head down and pressing your chest into the water, your hips will be lifted to the surface of the water which results in a level, balanced position. By having students practice this over short distances with a very easy kick, they can get the feel for the difference between the two positions. When performing this skill, encourage students to lift their head forward just enough to get air. This will help them experience how their body will become unbalanced as their hips and legs sink. After taking a breath, they should re-balance by looking back down at the bottom of the pool (hiding the head). At the same time, they should also press their upper torso and head into the water as a single unit. When done correctly, they should feel that the water is supporting their hips and legs. An effective instructional tip is to have students imagine they have a laser light coming out of the top of their head. If they are perfectly balanced, the light from this laser will hit the wall at the far end of their lane just above the water.

Figure 10.1   Balanced Body Position (head up and down)

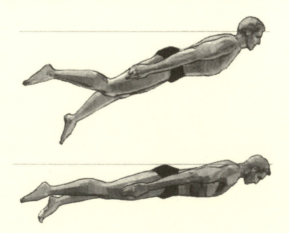

Body Position: Instructional Cues

- Hide your head
- Where is your laser light pointing?
- Press your chest into the water
- Look at the bottom of the pool
- Feel the water lift your hips
- Float level

The Flutter Kick

The flutter kick is the leg action that is used in the freestyle stroke. It consists of a shallow kick, 12-18 inches deep, which originates from the hip. The propulsion comes from the downward portion of the leg kick. The legs bend slightly on the downward portion of the kick (the propulsive phase) and then straighten on the upward portion (the recovery phase). The ankles should remain loose and flex throughout the kick. The leg action is very similar to the action of gently kicking a soccer ball in the air repetitively.

The most common error beginners' make in learning the flutter kick is to move the legs in a bicycling motion. This movement will hinder forward propulsion and the achievement of a balanced body position. As a general rule, it is better too kick too little than too big. As students learn the balanced body position, the need for a hard kick diminishes.

In teaching the flutter kick, have students begin in the "hide the head" position with their hands at their side. Have them begin by kicking short distances in order to get a feel for the kick. As they feel the need to breathe, they can lift their head, breathe, and then re-balance. If students are having difficulty practicing the kick in the balanced position, you can add kickboards which will enable them to focus their efforts solely on the kick. You can also provide fins to students who are having difficulty generating forward motion. Fins will allow them to experience what adequate propulsion from their legs feels like and are usually only needed for a short period of time. Fins are also a very effective tool for correcting the bicycle kick which causes inefficient forward movement. This is best accomplished by having students' kick in a stationary position with their hands grasping the side of the pool. As they practice this drill, it is important for them to keep their head in the water, looking at the bottom of the pool. They can simply raise their heads as needed to breathe.

Instructional Cues: Flutter Kick

- Kick from the hips
- Loose ankles
- Bend knees on the downward kick
- Small, shallow kick
- Keep legs and feet in the water
- Stay balanced

Breathing

The key to breathing comfortably lies in learning to "roll" the body towards the surface. The entire body should roll as a single unit with the shoulders, abdomen, and hips all rotating like a log. The instructional cue "roll to the air" will guide students toward the proper movement without lifting the head. Many swimmers are taught to turn their head to breathe, and in doing so they discover they need to lift their head in order to get air. As the head is lifted, the body will naturally come out of balance and the swimmer will feel as if they are swimming "uphill."

The first step in learning to breathe correctly is to master balancing on your side with the bottom arm extended. This is the same balancing position on the abdomen that was described earlier only now the student is on their side. Begin by having the students roll onto their side with their bottom arm extended and continue to roll slightly toward their back until their face is exposed and they can breathe comfortably. This is called the "sweet spot." The precise angle at which each student must roll past 90 degrees is different for each individual. A novice swimmer will probably have to roll more toward their back. Students should not rotate all the way to their back and they should strive to keep their head down, in line with their body. Remind them of their laser light! The palm of their hand should be facing the bottom of the pool and their arm should be slightly underwater.

The kick should be performed while the student is on their side and their focus should be on pressing in on the bottom armpit. In addition, it is important to minimize the gap between the head and the shoulder and to try to keep most of the upper arm out of the water. Encourage your students to "stretch" as tall as possible from their fingertips of their toes. Short trips across the pool with both individualized and group-directed feedback after each lap is an effective way to teach this skill. The addition of fins can assist those students who are still struggling because they increase propulsion.

The Sweet Spot: Instructional Cues

- Lean in on bottom armpit
- Show the upper arm
- Small gap between head and shoulder
- Stretch from fingers to toes

Figure 10.2   Side Line Balanced Position—"The Sweet Spot"

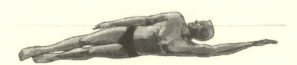

- Keep bottom arm underwater
- Laser light pointing at far end of pool
- Look straight up
- Keep head in line with body

The next progression is to rotate the head downward, placing the face in the water, and then recovering to the face up position while remaining on the side. This drill serves as a lead-up to learning to breathe without raising the head. The student should begin in the nose-up position, kicking in the sweet spot, and pressing the upper torso into the water. In addition, they should focus on pressing the back of the head into the shoulder of the bottom arm while their face is turned upward for air. After several yards, have the students turn their heads and look down at the bottom of the pool. By repeating this cycle several times, your students should begin to feel comfortable and balanced in both the nose up and nose down positions.

Instructional Cues: Nose Up-Nose Down

- Pause and balance in each position
- Look at bottom of pool or ceiling
- Stay on your side as you rotate your head
- Show your upper arm
- Nose up—back of head on bottom shoulder
- Nose down—chin on bottom shoulder

The Armstroke

The arms play an important role not only in lengthening the body, but also in providing the anchor points for propulsion. The longer the vessel, the more speed it will carry, and the arms play a major role in lengthening the human vessel. The

Figure 10.3   Nose Up-Nose Down on Side

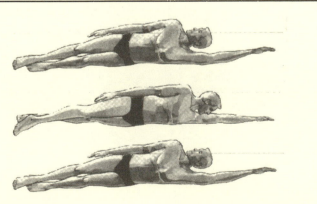

key instructional cue for prompting your students to achieve this increased length is "swim tall."

"Stop . . . Stop . . . Switch" is a very effective drill to learn the proper arm stroke. It begins in the nose upside-balanced position (the first stop). The head is then turned downward so that the student is looking at the bottom of the pool while still remaining on the side (the second stop). While still on the side, move the rear arm and place it in front of the head. When the student sees their hand entering the water they execute the "switch." This is performed by pulling the lead hand under the water while simultaneously rolling the entire body to the opposite side to a nose up position. The recovering arm then continues to keep the vessel long by reaching in front of the body. The "stop" always refers to the head position and the "switch" occurs when the body is rolled to the other side. Students should pause on their side to balance before repeating the movement in the other direction. During the roll, it is important that the student's face turns with their body to the nose up position. Students can ingrain this pattern by repeating the phrase "stop . . . stop . . . switch" and as this timing is perfected, stu-

Figure 10.4   Stop . . . Stop . . . Switch Drill

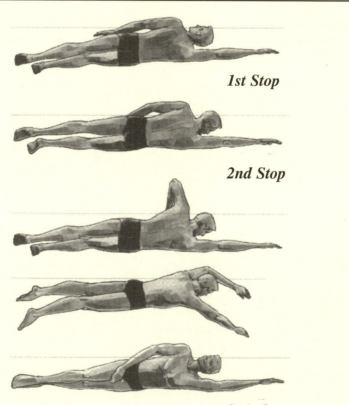

1st Stop

2nd Stop

Switch

dents should feel an acceleration which is caused by the surge of each switch. Although the stops are deliberate, the switch should be executed quickly.

Instructional Cues: Stop . . . Stop . . . Switch

• Say "Stop . . . Stop . . . Switch" as you execute the drill
• Deliberate "stop"
• Quick "switch"
• Keep your laser light in place
• Roll the body like a log
• Extend the arm forward in line with your body
• Begin stroking with lead hand when other arm enters water in front of head

Common errors:

• Omitting the second stop (head down)
• Student's lead hand begins to pull as soon as their trail arm begins to recover

Putting It All Together: The Freestyle Stroke

Once the previous drills have been mastered, students can now progress to combining these skills into a smooth, seamless, freestyle stroke. Begin by having your students' practice the "hips rotating with the armstroke sequence" for short distances. The goal is to get them to feel as if they are "skating" from one hip to the other while practicing the timing of the arm stroke. Ask them to imagine that their entire body, from the lead arm to the toes, is a blade on a speed skate. By keeping their head "hidden" and feeling the pressure transfer from their armpit to their chest, they should feel the sensation of swimming downhill!

Once students are comfortable with the timing of the arms and body rotation, they can add the breathing component by allowing their head to roll with the body. The inhalation phase occurs when their face is exposed to the surface. As their lead arm begins to stroke under the body, they should exhale forcefully as their arm begins to come out of the water. This prepares them for the next breath as the head rolls with the body.

FOCUS ON FITNESS

There are two simple games that students can do either individually or in a group setting that are fun, effective at promoting fitness, and reinforce the key principles of swimming.

Swimming Golf

This game involves swimming a predetermined distance, as fast as possible, with the fewest strokes possible. The "swimming golf score" is the sum of the time and stroke count. If the time to swim a given distance is 45 seconds, and the number of

Figure 10.5   Skating on Your Side

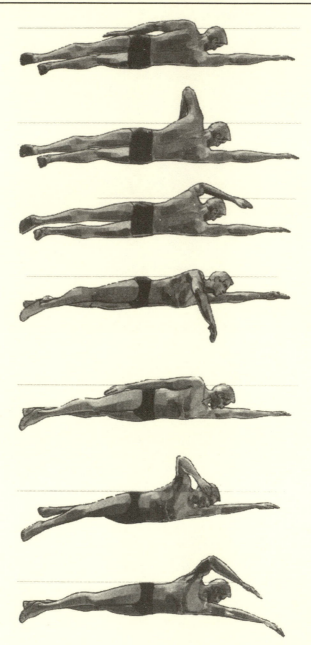

strokes is 43 (a stroke is every time the hand enters the water), then the swimming golf score is 88. In order to lower the score, the average swimmer will speed up their stroke rate (SR). However, in gaining a few seconds of speed they may take too many strokes and their score can actually increase. Encourage students to try to lower their score by becoming more efficient by increasing the distance they cover with each stroke (increase their stroke length). Swimming speed is a product of both stroke rate and stroke length, and novice swimmers usually only focus on stroke rate. The challenge is to try to lower the score using the most efficient combination of the two. If you have a large class, have your students swim four, 50-yard distances by leaving at 10-second intervals. Instruct them to count their own strokes and have a student with a stopwatch call out their times. Each student then listens for their time and adds the time, in seconds, to their stroke count. Allow them to rest for 2 minutes once the last swimmer finishes. Challenge them to lower their score on each of the remaining three, 50-yard swims.

As students will learn, the fastest swimmer may not always have the best golf score. In addition, it is recommended that the teacher de-emphasize competition. If students choose to compete, the teacher can create swimming golf handicaps, based on swimming ability, to equalize the competition. The real value of the initial golf score is that it serves as an initial self-assessment for each student and provides them with an individualized method for tracking their progress.

Stroke Eliminators

Stroke Eliminators challenges students to swim using fewer strokes. Begin by having your students swim one length of the pool at a comfortable pace and have them count their strokes. Repeat this 4 times, with a brief rest after each length, in order to determine their average number of strokes. We will call this number "N." The next step consists of having them swim a three-length sequence in which the first length has a stroke count of N+1, the second length at N, and the final length at N-1. For example, if the N is 12, the stroke counts for each length would be 13, 12, and 11. The challenge for the student is to repeat this three-length sequence several times while maintaining the same time.

There are a great variety of activities that can be created using "stroke count" and "time" as the key variables. Holding one of these two variables constant while attempting to reduce the other is the desired goal, and distances can be adjusted periodically to keep the activity interesting.

SAMPLE LESSON PLAN

This lesson is designed for 20-25 high school students who have basic swimming skills and have already learned the basic balancing drills. The required equipment includes a stopwatch and 6 lanes.

Scope of the Lesson: Introduction to the "Stop . . . Stop . . . Switch" Drill

Sequence of the Lesson (45 minute class)

1. Warm-up—review lead balance drills (10 minutes).
   - Four students per lane. Practice one length of head lead balance (kicking on stomach, "hiding head," with hands at side). Raise head forward to breathe and re-balance.
   - Alternate with one length of side line balance in "sweet spot" (arm in front, face up, work on finding "sweet spot," and showing top arm). This should be done on both sides.
   - Teacher observes and provides individual feedback.
2. Provide group-directed feedback on your observations. Practice perfect length of side line balance (3 minutes).
3. Review and model the "Stop . . . Stop . . . Switch" (SSS) drill (5 minutes).
4. Practice one length of SSS Drill with students leaving one after another in their lane. Teacher looks for a student that performs it well to demonstrate (2 minutes).
5. Selected student demonstrates the SSS drill with the teacher highlighting the key instructional cues (3 minutes).
6. Students repeat single lengths, stopping at each end, for both individual and group-directed feedback (10 minutes).
7. Pair up students and have them observe their partner for two lengths. Students provide peer-feedback to one another. Switch roles after two lengths (8 minutes).
8. Provide effective closure: review the lesson, its relevance, and the instructional cues (2-3 minutes).

Major Skill Theme

"Stop . . . Stop . . . Switch" Drill

Instructional Cues

- Start in a balanced position
- Deliberate pause at each "stop"
- Make the "switch" brisk
- Roll the body like a log
- Roll the head to the air
- Feel a "surge" after the switch
- Lead arm extended until other hand enters water
- Replace lead arm with other arm to lengthen body
- Transfer press from armpit to chest to armpit during switch
- Pull body over hand that is stroking underwater

Teaching Styles

* Command Style for initial demonstration
* Individualized Instruction/Practice Centered (instructor rotates from student to student as students practice SSS Drill)
* Peer/ Reciprocal assessment utilized by students as they observe one another swim

TERMINOLOGY

Balance: Floating on the surface of the water so that all parts of the body are supported equally.

Freestyle: The most commonly used swimming stroke, also called the front crawl. The fastest of the four competitive strokes.

Hand Lead Balance: Balancing in the water on the side, with the bottom arm extended forward, and the other arm at the side.

Head Lead Balance: Balancing in the water, on either the stomach or back, with the arms at the side.

Hiding the Head: Keeping the head in line with the torso by looking down rather than forward while swimming. Only the upper third of the head is above the water.

Kickboards: Styrofoam boards that are used for kicking.

Lane Lines: Plastic flotation devices on a line that run the length of a pool and divide the lanes.

Masters Swim Clubs: An organization of adult swimmers which is regulated by a national governing body.

Pace Clock: A large clock located at one end of a pool which enables swimmers to determine their times.

Paddles: Flat, rectangular devices made of plastic and strapped to the hands to place additional stress on the arms.

Pull Bouys: Styrofoam devices that fit between the upper thighs and support the legs and allow the swimmer to focus on the arms for propulsion.

Scull: To sweep the hands and arms back and forth in a motion that results in propulsion.

Skating: The action of rotating the hips from side to side in coordination with the armstroke.

Stroke Cycle: The completion of the arm movement through a complete stroke (e.g. each time the right hand enters the water equals one stroke cycle).

Stroke Eliminators: A training technique that establishes a base number of strokes per length (N) and challenges the swimmer to complete lengths with a stroke count greater than or less than N.

Stroke Length: The distance a swimmer's body travels during each stroke cycle.

Stroke Rate: The speed at which the arms rotate.

Sweet Spot: The balance point, in which the swimmer is on their side, looking up at the ceiling, and their head is in line with their torso. This is the position in which the balance drills begin and end.

Swimming Golf: A fun activity in which a swimming golf score is achieved. The score is the sum of the number of strokes taken over a particular distance and the time it takes to swim the distance.

Swimming Tall: Always keeping one arm in front of your head as you swim in order to lengthen the bodyline. This is accomplished by waiting to begin the stroke with the lead arm until the hand on the recovering arm is entering the water in front of the head.

SELECTED READINGS

Brems, M. (1998). *A Fit Swimmer: 120 Workouts and Training Tips*. Chicago, IL: NTC/Contemporary Publishing.

Callison, B. (1998). *Swim For Life*. Barcal.

Guzman, R. (1998). *Swimming Drills for Every Stroke*. Champaign, IL: Human Kinetics Publishers.

Hines, E. (1998). *Fitness Swimming*. Champaign, IL: Human Kinetics Publishers.

Katz, J. et al (1993). *Swimming For Total Fitness: A Progressive Aerobic Program*. Garden City, NY: Doubleday.

Langendorfer, S. & Brya, L. (1995). *Aquatic Readiness: Developing Water Competence in Young Children*. Champaign, IL: Human Kinetics.

Laughlin, T. (1997). *Total Immersion: the Revolutionary Way to Swim Better, Faster, and Easier*. Fireside.

Leonard, J. (1994). *Rookie Coaches Swimming Guide*. Champaign, IL: Human Kinetics.

Lepore, M., Gayle G. & Stevens, S. (1998). *Adaptive Aquatics Programming: A Professional Guide*. Champaign, IL: Human Kinetics.

Tarpinian, S. (1996). *The Essential Swimmer*. New York: Lyons Press.

Whiten, P. (1994). *The Complete Book of Swimming*. New York: Random House.

SPORT SPECIFIC ORGANIZATIONS

United States Swimming
One Olympic Plaza
Colorado Springs, CO 80909
(719) 578-4578
FAX (719) 578-4669
http://www.usa-swimming.org

American Swimming Coaches Association
304 S.E. 20th Street
Fort Lauderdale, FL 33316
(305) 462-6267
FAX (305) 462-6280
http://www.swimmingcoach.org

Appendix

National Organizations
National Collegiate Athletic Association
       700 W. Washington Ave.
       PO Box 6222
       Indianapolis IN 46206-6222

National Association of State and High School Athletic Association
       7 South Dearborn St.
       Chicago, IL 60603

Sport Specific Organizations
Running
Road Runners Club of America
       National Office
       1150 South Washington, Suite 250
       Alexandria, VA 22314

Cycling
United States Cycling Federation
       1750 Boulder St.
       Colorado Springs, CO 80909

Volleyball
USA Volleyball
       715 S. Circle Dr.
       Colorado Springs, CO 80910

Index

ABOUT THE AUTHOR AND CONTRIBUTORS

RAYMOND J. BOSSE was the Head Coach of both men's and women's swimming at the United States Military Academy for 13 years. He also instructs swimming as a coach with *Total Immersion*, a highly regarded learn to swim program known around the world.

LAWRENCE F. BUTLER is Associate Professor, Department of Physical Education, United States Military Academy at West Point.

KAREN Y. PECK is now an instructor and athletic trainer at the United States Military Academy at West Point and is the course director for tennis.